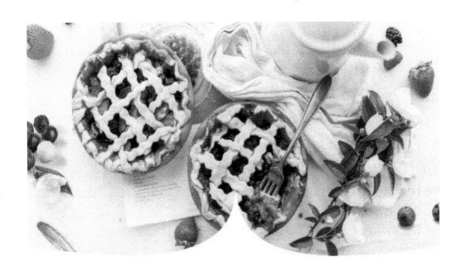

Sirtfood Diet

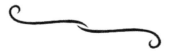

"We are what we eat"

Adele Bayles

Table of Contents

BY ADELE BAYLES

INTRODUCTION...7
The top 20 sirtfoods...9
   Bird eye chili..9
   Buckwheat...9
   Capers..10
   Celery..10
   Cocoa...10
   Extra virgin oil..11
   Coffee..11
   Green tea...11
   Kale..12
   Lovage..12
   Medjool dates...12
   Parsley...13
   Red chicory...13
   Rocket..13
   Red wine..14
   Soy...14
   Strawberries..14
   Turmeric..15
   Walnuts...15
   Red onions..15
Sirtuins...18
   Benefits of sirtuins..18
Sirti Activator..21
BLUE ZONES: Does the sirt diet extend life?......................22
Blue zones...23
Sirtfood diet program and best ways to maintain results..........25
Kitchen measurement conversion chart.............................30

SIRTFOOD DIET RECIPES..31

Breakfast recipes...**32**

   Buckwheat porridge...33

   Kale with scrambled egg.....................................35

   Waffles..37

   Kale omelet with smoked salmon......................39

   Broccoli salad..41

   Apple cinnamon omelet.....................................43

   Mushroom kale with frittata..............................45

   Citrus salad with kale..47

   Berries arugula with salad.................................50

   Granola buckwheat...52

   Apple cakes..55

   Salmon with scrambled egg...............................57

   Spinach with egg scramble................................59

   Veggie omelet..61

   Coconut porridge...64

   Swiss card with chickpea...................................66

   Pak choi stir fry with prawns.............................68

   Arugula salad with nuts.....................................70

   Sweet potato fries with avocado dip..................72

   Salmon with capers...74

Lunch recipes..**76**

   Mediterranean pizza..77

   Shrimp skillet with kale.....................................79

   Kale salad with ginger and carrot.....................81

   Salmon burger with spicy sauce........................83

   Creamy kale salad with raspberry.....................85

   Bacon with sweet potato salad..........................87

   Lettuce wraps..89

   Brunoise salad...92

   Melon salad with ham..94

   Cauliflower pizza..96

   Roasted pumpkin salad......................................98

   Chicken rolls..101

   Caesar chicken...103

Pork carnitas..105
Meatloaf...107
Carrot salad..109
Chicken curry...111
Chicken flautas...113
Tuna stuffed avocado..116
Chilli corn carne...118
Zoodles with shrimp florentine..120
Tomato salsa..122
Shakshuka...124
Braised cabbage...126
Indian shrimp curry...128
Sweet potato hash...130
Cauliflower fritters..132
Date and bacon appetizer..134
Ensalada rusa...136
Shrimp with scrambled eggs..138

Dinner recipes..140
Veggie stir-fry with soba noodle..141
Asparagus with prawn tagliatelle..143
Grilled vegetables..145
Spicy potato curry..147
Stuffed eggplant..149
Broccoli with chicken...151
Toasted pine nuts with green kale.......................................153
Mushroom with bok choy..155
Lamb chops with crispy kale...157
Peanut curry with broccoli and tofu.....................................160
Steak salad...162
Lettuce wraps...165
Sauteed chicory greens..168
Cauliflower fried rice..170
Spicy meatballs...173
Pumpkin pasta...176
Chorizo potatoes..178
Basil with tomato sauce...180

Chorizo with rigatoni pasta..................................... 182
Kale super salad...184
Surf and turf... 186
Garlic lemon scallops...188
Teriyaki tempeh... 190
Okonomiyaki.. 193
Keema curry.. 195
Beef burrito.. 198
Nasi goreng...200
Beef rendang... 203
Fried fish vegetable... 206
Fish fingers.. 209
Soups recipes... 211
Lentil soup... 212
Kale with bean soup... 215
Broccoli courgette soup.. 217
Carrot and pumpkin soup...................................... 219
Creamy potato soup..221
Shrimp garlic butter soup......................................223
Sweet potato soup... 225
Turmeric soup with lentil...................................... 227
Harira soup.. 229
Carrot and beetroot soup...................................... 231
Snacks recipes..233
Baking powder biscuits... 234
Chocolate granola bites...237
Chocolate muffins.. 240
Peanut brittle... 242
Snickers bars..244
Pizza crackers... 247
Buttery pretzels..249
Bark snowflakes..252
Peanut butter cookies.. 254
Dessert recipes...256
Blueberry muffins...257
Cinnamon apple wraps...259

Strawberry mousse..261

Vanilla ice cream coconut cream.........................263

Cheesecake in jar...265

Blueberry chocolate cake....................................267

Red velvet cake..269

Espresso brownies..272

Pumpkin roll..275

Pecan pie...277

Juice & drinks recipes......................................279

Green tea matcha...280

Celery juice..282

Orange kale..284

Cucumber apple juice...286

Green lemon juice..288

Watermelon juice...290

Vinaigrette juice..292

Pineapple juice..294

Strawberry juice..296

Bulletproof coffee...298

7 days meal plan...300

TIPS: Popular questions and answers on sirtfood diet.............. 303

DISCLAIMER..305

Thank you!...306

INTRODUCTION

Your diet is crucial for your survival. A bad diet will not provide the necessary nutrients needed for long life. A healthy diet will optimally invigorate your body and help prevent diseases caused by nutritional deficiencies. A healthy diet will also help in speeding up recovery to injuries (internal or external).

The Sirtfood diet is a diet based on Sirtfoods. Sirtfoods is a recently discovered group of food that helps metabolism and reduces cell inflammation for better health.

Some diet books are written to primarily help people with weight loss but those types of diet plans might cause nutritional deficiencies. Here, you will learn how to eat healthily and have a good lifestyle change. Weight loss is not the primary goal and effect of the Sirtfood diet. Sirtfood diet will enable you to consume some of your favorite foods and drinks while losing weight at the same time.

The main aim of the Sirtfood diet is to help the body activate the sirtuin genes properly. The sirtuin genes have numerous functions in the body. They protect specific cells from dying and increase metabolism rate.

All information in this book have been well researched, and my experience as a diet book writer should help remove any doubt you might have on any information. My interest in the enzymology of sirtuins was a major reason for writing this book. As you read on you will discover that I accurately explained how sirtuins help in regulating a person's life spans. My explanation will enable anybody with limited knowledge in biology to understand the science of sirtuins.

The Sirtfood diet was the 7th most googled diet in 2019. The Sirtfood diet is increasing in popularity, but many people still don't properly understand how it works.

People who understand sustainability still have fears about it but there is no need to worry about sustainability. This is because even celebrities like Adele Adkins (singer), David Haye (boxer), and Ben Ainslie (Olympic gold medalist) have directly and indirectly attested to the sustainability of the Sirtfood diet with regular exercise.

Follow the simple steps and recipes in this book, and you will surely have long term results.

The book has been divided into three sections. All sections will reveal specific information on Sirtfoods and Sirtuins activating compounds (SAC) that no other diet book will tell. The first section explicitly explains Sirtfoods and how the Sirtfood diet works.

The benefits and surprising characteristics of the top 20 Sirtfoods are also explained in the first section. The second section extensively describes the benefits of the sirtuin gene in the human body and why Sirtfoods properly activate it.

The third section is essential because it's the section where all Sirtfoods recipes and diet plans are described. This section also explains why the diet of people living in the five blue zones helps them live longer than the average human.

All sections are relevant and connected, so it is advisable to read all without skipping any.

For best results, every step, advice, and recipe in this book must be followed accordingly. Any deviation will be counter-productive to getting a new and positive lifestyle change.

THE TOP 20 SIRTFOODS

Here are the Top 20 Sirtfoods you need to know

Bird Eye Chili

This is mostly grown in east Africa and Southeast Asia. Its scientific name is capsicum annum which is the Latin for 'bird eye'. This particular chili pepper is scorching and has high amounts of capsaicin. Capsaicin is a sirtuin activating compound SAC. It helps in boosting metabolism and also reduces insulin spikes in diabetics.

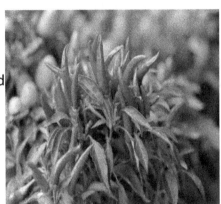

Buckwheat

This is a plant food very common in Asia It is a short and stocky shrub with white flowers. Buckwheat is usually processed into grains or granules. It is cooked like rice in most regions. The nutritional benefits of the buckwheat include; regulation of blood sugar and supply of dietary fiber.

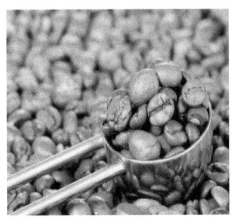

Capers

These are the immature flower buds of the caper bush, which are usually grown in the Mediterranean. They are mostly pickled or salted for preservation because they are low in carb and fat. They are rich in vitamin K.

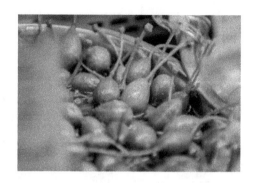

Celery

This is amongst the oldest cultivated plants. Celery has long fibrous roots that taper into leaves. It is a good source of antioxidants, but it should not be eaten in excess because of its salt content.

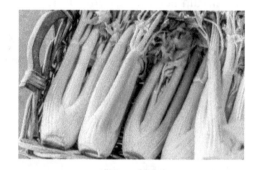

Cocoa

This is a very popular crop. It is fermented or roasted as cacao beans. Cocoa contains many SACs that helps the body stay healthy. It also helps with weight control.

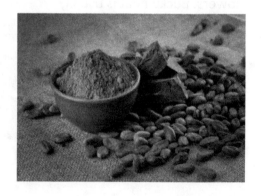

Extra Virgin Oil

This made from the purest, cold-pressed olives. This oil is the best for cooking as it is without being blended with any other processed oil. Cooking only with extra-virgin
olive oil helps in reducing the risk of heart disease.

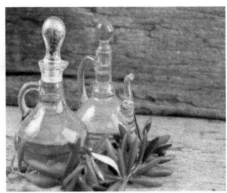

Coffee

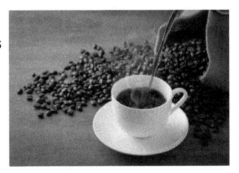

This is a popular drink that is made from roasted coffee beans. Coffee contains lots of SACs, but it shouldn't be taken in excess.

Green Tea

This drink originates from China. The buds and leaves of the green tea plant are processed like black teas. The Green Tea helps in weight loss increases the metabolism rate, thereby increasing fat loss.

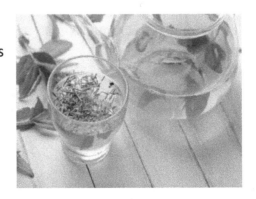

Kale

This originates from the Mediterranean. It is an edible cabbage. Kale is loaded with antioxidants and SACs like and just like the kaempferol, it helps in lowering excess cholesterol in the body.

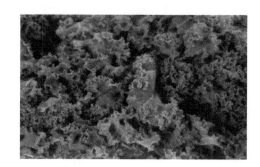

Lovage

Lovage is a perennial crop grown in southern Europe. The leaves of the Lovage plant are generally used as herbs, the seeds used as a spice, and the roots are used as
vegetables. Lovage contains SACs that helps for efficient digestion.

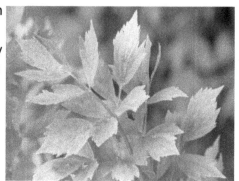

Medjool Dates

This is a vibrant and caramel like fruit from the palm family. It is also called date palm or date. It is full of natural sugars and contains a high amount of fiber.

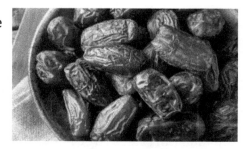

Parsley

This is a flowering plant that is cultivated as a vegetable and herb. Parsley is cultivated in the central and eastern Mediterranean. Parsley contains anti-bacterial properties and helps in regulating blood pressure.

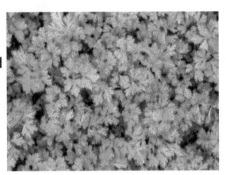

Red Chicory

This is cultivated for its leaves and is eaten raw as salads. It is a good source of prebiotic fiber insulin. It aids bowel movement and may promote weight loss.

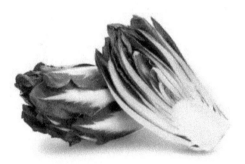

Rocket

This is also known as roquette. It is an English leaf used in salads. It is loaded with vitamin A, C, and K. Rocket contains glucosinolates, which help the body against cancer.

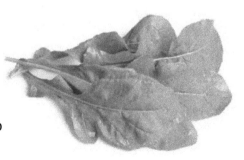

Red Wine

This is a famous wine made from dark grapes. Red wine contains (antioxidants resveratrol). Resveratrol prevents inflammations and blood clotting. The best red wine is the 'pinot noir.'

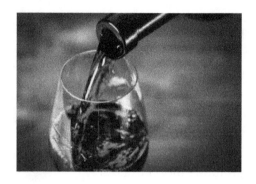

Soy

Soy comes from soybeans. Soybeans are common in East Asia. It is consumed as a form of plant protein. It contains SACS that helps in lowering excessive cholesterol.

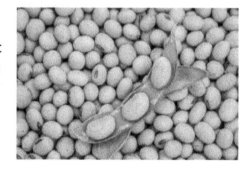

Strawberries

Strawberries are popular fruits that are packed with vitamin C and antioxidants. Strawberries also help in lowering blood pressure and excessive cholesterol.

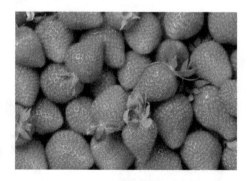

Turmeric

This is a flowering plant whose roots are used as a spice. It contains lots of SACs that helps in reducing inflammation and improving skin quality.

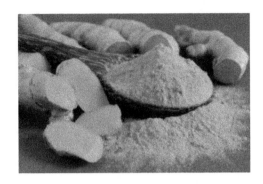

Walnuts

This is the edible seed of a drupe. Walnuts also contain a high level of antioxidants. Walnuts help in weight control and in managing diabetes (blood sugar level).

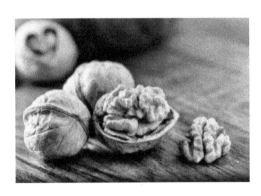

Red Onions

They are widely used in the culinary arts. They are usually bigger than the normal onions and have high eye-watering quality. They help in boosting bone density and digestive health.

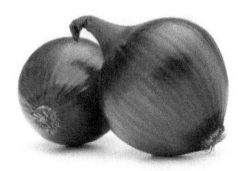

In addition to the Top 20 Sirt Foods, the following foods will also help in activating sirtuins:

Fruits

- Blackcurrant
- Blackberries
- Black Plums
- Apple
- Goji Berries
- Raspberries
- Black Grapes
- Kumquat

Vegetables

- Asparagus
- Chinese Cabbage
- Green Beans
- Shallot
- Artichokes
- White Onions

Dried Fruits

- Pistachios
- Sunflower Seeds
- Peanuts
- Chestnuts
- Chia Seeds

Cereals

- Quinoa
- Wholemeal Flour
- White Beans
- Fava Beans

Aromatic Herbs And Spices

- Ginger
- Chives
- Dried Oregano
- Dill
- Peppermint
- Dried Sage Thyme

Drink

- White Tea
- Black Tea

SIRTUINS

There are seven (7) sirtuins in the human cell. One can be found in the cytoplasm, three in the nucleus and mitochondria each. Sirtuins are part of the 60,000 cellular proteins in the human body.

Sirtuins are also called 'guardians of the genome'. They belong to a class of Nicotinamide Adenine Dinucleotide-consuming enzyme (NAD+enzyme). The NAD+ enzyme is made up of two nucleotides and is the basis of DNA. They play a vital role in metabolism.

Some polyphenols like Resveratrol can be found in many Sirtfoods. They also play vital roles in boosting metabolism and improving digestive issues. Resveratrol can be found in Sirtfoods-for instance: red wine and turmeric.

All benefits of sirtuins will be explained in subsequent pages.

BENEFITS OF SIRTUINS

Inflammation Reduction in the Heart

Heart infections or inflammations are caused by toxic particles in the air, bacteria, or virus. Sirtuins help in protecting the heart and reduce the risk of inflammation or myocarditis.

Scaling Up Cardio Protection

Strawberries and chocolates are two of the best Sirtfoods for boosting cardioprotection. With regular exercise and an increase in the consumption of Sirtfoods, the quality of heart muscles is increased.

Inflammation Reduction in the Intestines

This is also known as colitis. Some infections in the intestine are caused when the immune system mistakenly attacks a harmless bacteria in the colon. Sirtuins activating foods serve as an anti-inflammatory diet that helps in maintaining long term gut inflammation.

Adipogenesis Reduction

This is related to insulin resistance syndrome. It also contributes to the increase in tissue mass, that could cause obesity. Sirtfoods like green tea help in reducing Adiopogenesis and leptin resistance.

Lipogenesis Reduction

Lipogenesis is the process of fat formation from excess carbohydrates. An unhealthy and high carb diet Lipogenesis helps in increasing and generally increases body weight and reduces muscle mass. But, an excellent Sirtfood-diet will activate sirtuins properly, reduce Lipogenesis, and increase muscle mass.

Scaling Up Mitochiondriogenesis

Mitochondria are essential because they perform cellular respiration. Sirtuins increase the rate at which mitochondria break down nutrients to energy.

Neurodegeneration Reduction

When sirtuin is properly activated, there will be a reduction in the risk of neuron-disease like Alzheimer's.

Scaling Up Fat Metabolism

One primary function of the liver is fat metabolism for blood sugar regulation. Sirtuins increase this rate and help in preventing excess liver fat.

Scaling Up Gluconeogenesis

This is the formation of glucose from non-carbohydrate carbon saturates. Sirtuins help the liver in performing Gluconeogenesis efficiently.

Lipid-Profile Reduction

The lipid profile is the same as blood fats. High levels of blood fats will increase the risk of heart and liver diseases. Sirtuins help in the management and reduction of excess blood fats.

Scaling Up Fatty Acid Utilization In Muscles

One of the primary functions of muscles is the oxidation of fatty acids into glucose. Sirtuin increases the rate at which fatty acids are oxidized in muscles.

Scaling Up Insulin Secretion

Insulin is produced by the pancreas and is used for the regulation of glucose metabolism. Sirtfoods like capers and celery help in boosting insulin sensitivity and secretions.

Reduction In The Risk Of Tumor Growth

The risk of cancer is reduced when we properly activate sirtuins by eating Sirtfoods. Vegetables like kale and lovage contain anti-inflammatory compounds that will regulate blood pressure and reduces the risk of tumor growth.

Sirti Activator

Heart

- ⬇ Inflammation
- ⬆ Cardioprotection

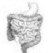

Intestine

- ⬇ Inflammation

Adipose

- ⬇ Adipogenesis
- ⬇ Lipogenesis
- ⬆ Mitocihondriogenesis

Brain/CNS

- ⬇ Neurodegeneration

Liver

- ⬆ Fat metabolism
- ⬆ Mitochondriogenesis
- ⬇ Gluconeogenesis
- ⬇ Lipid profiles

Skeletal Muscle

- ⬆ Mitochondriogenesis
- ⬆ Fatty-acid utilization
- ⬆ Insulin action

Pancreas

- ⬆ Insuline secretion

Tumor

- ⬇ Cancer growth

✗ 21

BLUE ZONES: DOES THE SIRT DIET EXTEND LIFE?

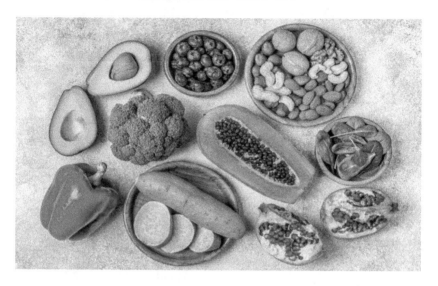

Aging is irreversible and inevitable. There is no way to halt the aging process, but there are many ways to extend it. There are two types of aging; **Unhealthy Aging and Healthy Aging.**

Unhealthy aging will create a reduction in life expectancy. This is caused by unhealthy diets, genetic mutations, and an unhealthy environment.

Healthy aging will create an increase in life expectancy. It happens when there is favorable interaction of a good environment, a healthy diet, and reduced genetic mutations. Healthy aging will be promoted further when there is an improvement in the quality of nutrient-sensing longevity genes.

Nutrient-sensing longevity genes help in regulating the life span of cells in the body. Sirtuin genes are the main members of this gene group. There are regions in the so-called blue zones.

The people living in these areas eat only foods rich in sirtuin-activating agents or compounds. Residents of the blue zones live healthier and longer than the average human. In no particular order, the regions in the blue zones will be explained in successive pages.

BLUE ZONES

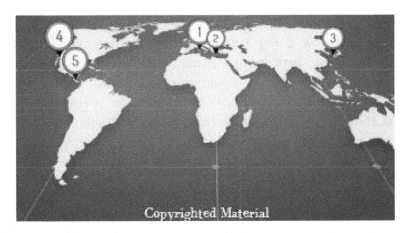

Ogiliastra, Sardinia

This is a mountainous highland in Italy. Ogiliastra boasts the highest population of centenarians in the world. Residents consume a low protein diet, associated with lower rates of diabetes and cancer. They also have good psychological well-being.

Ikaria, Greece

This is a small island in Greece. Here, the middle-age mortality rate is meager, and the percentage of people over 80 is higher than in most regions in Europe. The healthy aging of people in this region is as a result of their Mediterranean diet, which is substantial in Sirt vegetables, fruits, and small amounts of dairy.

Okinawa, Japan

Okinawa is the largest island in the archipelago in the south of Japan. Here, they eat until they are 80% full. This means only foods with low energy density will be consumed. They eat Sirtfoods with a high amount of carotenoids and low calories, which help them to age well.

Loma Linda, California

The community in Loma Linda has the highest population of Seventh-day Adventists in the world. Residents have very high life-expectancy because the community advocates vegetarianism and discourages the consumption of tobacco, beverages, and alcohol. They follow only a biblical diet full of Sirtfoods grown in the Mediterranean.

Nicoya Peninsula, Costa Rica

This is the cape region in Central America. Here, they have the lowest consumption of processed foods in the world. Nicoya has the world's lowest rate of middle-age mortality and the second-highest concentration of centenarians. Their secret lies in their nutrient-dense diet with a low glycemic index and high fiber content.

Tropical fruits, beans, and corn are popular foods in Nicoya. Nicoyans have deep spiritual habits, and they also engage in regular, low-intensity physical activities.

You will notice that residents of the blue zones eat less processed foods, small amounts of meat and fish. The reason is that their Sirtfood diet promotes mostly plant-based foods that provide them with a very long and healthy life.

SIRTFOOD DIET PROGRAM AND BEST WAYS TO MAINTAIN RESULTS

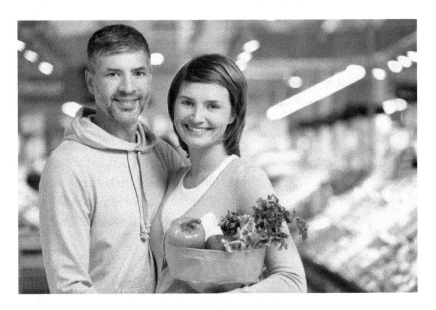

Dieting is the practice of consuming food in an organized manner to efficiently reduce, maintain, and in some cases, increase body weight.

The right diet program will ultimately help in reducing the risk of cancer, improve heart health, prevent stroke, increase the quality of bones, and improve brain functions.

Most diet programs like the Sirtfood diet program are designed to enable dieters to eat more vegetables, fruits, and low-fat dairy products. Contrary to popular opinion, diet programs are not only created for people looking to lose weight. Diet programs can also be used by people who want to maintain their body weight, shape, and health. No-one will tell you this, but, the truth is; you will spend more on a random diet plan than on a well-planned diet like the Sirtfood diet program.

The Sirtfood program has two phases. These two phases will be described in subsequent pages.

Phase 1: 7 days

This phase is also called the 'hyper-success' phase. Here, you are expected to lose a minimum of 7lbs in 7 days. Most people are usually under the impression that losing 7lbs in 7 days is impossible, but it is possible. The only thing is when you lose weight that fast, lots of it will be water, and only a small quantity will be actual body fat.

In this seven (7) days-phase, you must reduce your intake of calorie to not more than 1000 calories. One Sirtfood rich-meal and three green juices must be taken per day for this calorie restriction phase to work. You can also eat snacks like chocolate bars during this period, but they must not be consumed in excess.

If you can't follow this type of calorie restriction for seven (7) days, then try to follow it for just three (3) days. Most first-time dieters might still feel light-headed during these three (3) days, but that's normal because it's an adaptation period for your body.

For the remaining four (4) days, calorie intake can be increased to not more than 1500 calories. The diet for the remaining four (4) days will include; 2 Sirtfood meals and 2 cups of green juices per day. Remember, this method is meant to be followed by those who can't sustain 1000 calorie intake for the first week.

If you feel you can sustain 1000 calorie intake for exactly seven (7) days, then do so. You must also avoid alcohol during phase 1. Coffee, Medjool date smoothie and Green-tea are drinks that could be ingested but not in excess.

Phase 2: 14 days

This is also known as 'the maintenance' phase. It lasts for a minimum of 14 days. Phase 2 must start immediately after phase 1 because any break between each phase would be counter-productive.

In phase 2, calorie restriction is not the aim, but you will still experience a continuous weight loss. For the 14 days, it is advisable to consume at most 3 Sirtfood-rich meals and 1 cup of green juice per day. Alcohol is also not allowed during this phase, but red wine can be consumed.

Red wine contains lots of SACs just like resveratrol, but you should not take it in excess. 2-3 glasses per week are enough. Also, unlike the phase 1, you will certainly not feel light-headed because, at this phase, your body could have adjusted to the diet change made.

Sirtfood diet program should be long term. It is advisable to increase the duration of phase 2 to three or more weeks. In order not to be counter-productive, exercise like the Pilate routine should become regular as your body gets used to the diet program. Physical activities will help you retain and efficiently tone muscle mass.

Regular hydration during phase 2 of the diet program is also essential because drinking enough water at the right time will help regulate blood sugar levels and improve metabolism. It will also allow the kidney and liver to function better.

The summary of the Sirtfood diet program is:

Phase 1

- During the 'hyper success' phase, reduce calories to not more than 1500 calories.
- Drink, at most, 2 cups of green juices per day

- Eat one Sirtfood-rich meal per day; (snacks like chocolate can be included in small amounts.)

Phase 2

- During the 'maintenance period,' calories intake per day should not be more than 3000 calories
- Consume three Sirtfood-rich meals and, at most, 2 cups of green juice per day. Snacks like chocolates, red wine can be added to meals too.
- Hydration and physical activities must increase.

Best Ways to Maintain Results

Completing both phases of the diet (minimum of 3 weeks) is not enough for the overall effect of the Sirtfood diet and the SACs to last.

Sirtfoods are not magical foods, and they don't work overnight. Patience is needed because the Sirtfood diet program is not meant to be a 'one-off' program. It is meant to be 'a way of life.'

You will know it is working when the diet becomes your lifestyle and friends and family commend you for your diet change and commitment.

Yes, the Sirtfood diet program is demanding, but in the long term, it will be worth it.

Three (3) ways to efficiently maintain results are:
- ➤ You have to consistently eat only Sirtfood-rich meals, green juices, and never relapse to your usual processed foods. Recipes for the best Sirtfood meals to follow will be included in the next chapter.
- ➤ Connect more with people who are also following the Sirtfood diet program to remove any feeling of loneliness during your diet journey. One reason many stop dieting is because they

don't have any other dieter to encourage them when they don't see changes.

➢ Scale-up weight loss-exercise and increase overall physical activity to allow all diet changes to work better. This will also help to reduce muscle weakness that might be felt because of calorie restriction.

Kitchen Measurement
Conversion Chart

1 teaspoon (TSP) = 5ml

1 tablespoon (TBSP) = 3 teaspoons = 15ml

2 tablespoons = 1 oz (1 fluid ounce) = 30ml

4 tablespoons = 1/4 cup = 60ml

5 tablespoons + 1 teaspoon = 1/3 cup = 80ml

1/2 cup = 8 tablespoons = 120ml

1 cup = 16 tablespoons = 240ml

1 Quart = 2 pints = 4 cups

1 gallon = 4 quarts = 16 cups

SIRTFOOD DIET RECIPES

Breakfast
Recipes

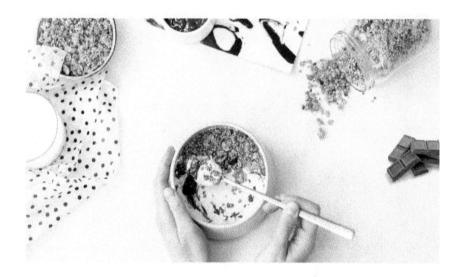

Adele Bayles

BUCKWHEAT PORRIDGE

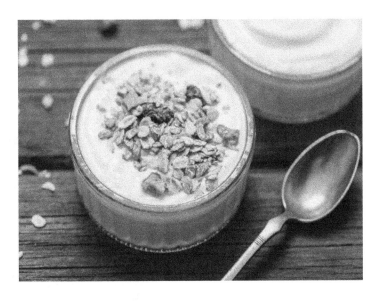

Buckwheat porridge is a portion of delicious comfort food that is rich in copper, zinc, and manganese. It's a complete protein that is loaded with all nine (9) essential amino acids and tons of fiber.

You can enjoy this breakfast meal by topping it up with cinnamon, fresh cinnamon, a splash of almond milk, and vanilla.

Enjoy!

PREP TIME: 6 mins
COOK TIME: 12 mins
TOTAL TIME: 18 mins
YIELD: 1 serving

NUTRITIONAL INFO

Calories: 142 cal | **Total fat:** 1.1 g | **Sodium:** 9.25 mg | **Sugar:** 0 g | **Vitamin A:** 0g | **Cholesterol:** 0 mg | **Carbohydrates:** 30.2 g | **Protein:** 4.3 g | **Vitamin C:** 0 mg

INGREDIENTS

- 1/2 cup of
- buckwheat groats, rinsed
- 1 cup of water

DIRECTIONS

- Add water and buckwheat groats into a small pot to medium-high heat.
- Bring it to a boil and reduce to a simmer.
- Use the lid to cover the pot and place the heat on low.
- Simmer for about 10 minutes, do not overcook. You can use a timer.
- Turn off the heat after 10 minutes.
- Do not open the lid and allow it to steam for another 5 minutes. Fluff with a fork.
- Serve and top with almond milk, cherries, a splash of vanilla, a drizzle of honey or maple syrup, and a dash of cinnamon.
- Enjoy.

KALE WITH SCRAMBLED EGG

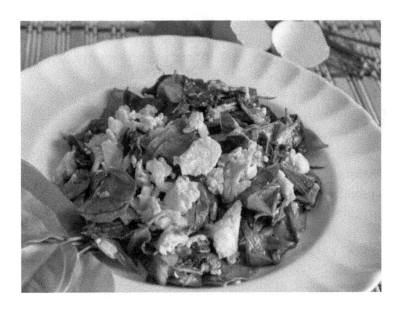

Kale with Scrambled egg is a quick, healthier breakfast made with fresh baby kale, and Parmesan cheese. It's the kind of recipe that can be ready within 15 minutes.

Fresh baby kale tastes fantastic with Parmesan cheese and eggs. You will get more vitamins, fiber, and minerals if you can eat this morning meal.

PREP TIME: 15 mins
COOK TIME: 0 mins
TOTAL TIME: 15 mins
YIELD: 1 serving

NUTRITIONAL INFO

Calories: 48 cal | **Total fat:** 1 g | **Saturated Fat:** 1/2 g | **Sodium:** 215 mg | **Sugar:** 1/2 g | **Vitamin A:** 500g | **Iron:** 1 mg | **Cholesterol:** 2 mg | **Carbohydrates:** 1/8 g | **Protein:** 7 g | **Vitamin C:** 1/2 mg

INGREDIENTS

- 0.3 cup of finely chopped yellow onion
- 0.4 cup of chopped fresh baby kale
- 0.6 teaspoon of garlic salt
- 1/2 cup of Egg Beaters
- 1 tablespoon of shredded parmesan cheese

DIRECTIONS

- Use cooking spray to spray large skillet.
- Place over medium heat and add onion.
- Cook until crisp-tender, for about 2 minutes.
- Add garlic, salt, and kale.
- Cook and stir until kale wilts, for another 1 minute.
- Add egg beaters and cook without stirring until the bottom and edges begin to set.
- Gently turn to scramble. Keep cooking until set.
- Top with cheese.
- Serve immediately and enjoy.

WAFFLES

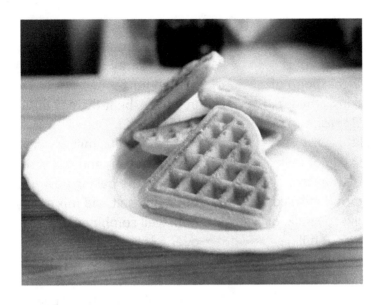

Waffles nutritional and preservative-free. They are extremely high in fiber and provide you with a complete protein from 100% vegetable sources. This recipe is built-up with high-quality ingredients that are so delicious and nutritious.

They are also fantastic for breakfast, and they can be perfect for dessert too. You can top with fruit and a dollop of whipped cream. You would love it! Add strawberries or berries to elevate it.

PREP TIME: 5 mins
COOK TIME: 10 mins
TOTAL TIME: 15 mins
YIELD: 1 serving

NUTRITIONAL INFO

Calories: 379 cal | **Total fat:** 17 g | **Saturated Fat:** 9 g | **Sodium:** 525 mg | **Sugar:** 18 g | **Vitamin A:** 905iu | **Iron:** 3.9 mg | **Cholesterol:** 243 mg | **Carbohydrates:** 62 g | **Protein:** 17 g | **Vitamin C:** 1/2 mg | **Potassium:** 538 mg | **Fiber:** 1 mg | **Calcium:** 268 mg

INGREDIENTS

- 1 large egg
- 1/2 cup of all purpose flour
- 1/2 teaspoon of baking powder
- 1/8 teaspoon of salt
- 1/2 cup of milk (you may use almond milk, cows milk, soy milk, or coconut milk)
- 1/4 teaspoon of vanilla extract
- 1 tablespoon of butter, melted
- 1 tablespoon of granulated sugar

DIRECTIONS

- Preheat waffle iron.
- Spray the iron with nonstick cooking spray or brush with melted butter.
- In a bowl, beat the egg until fluffy.
- Add the vanilla, milk, sugar, melted butter, and mix well.
- Whisk in the baking powder, flour, and salt and mix gently until well combined. Do not over mix it.
- Pour the batter on the iron. Then close it.
- You might have too much batter depending on the size of your waffle maker. So if so, use the little bit of remaining batter to make a second smaller waffle.
- Cook the waffle until no more steam comes out or waffle iron's indicator light shows that cooking is complete.
- The waffle should be crisp and golden brown.
- Bring out the waffle from the iron using a pair of tongs.
- Serve yourself & enjoy it immediately.

KALE OMELET WITH SMOKED SALMON

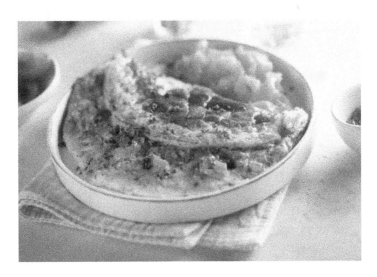

This kind of recipe is a delicious, tasty, and healthy meal that is easy to prepare. Getting enough of Kale Omelet with Smoked Salmon recipe will keep your tissues strong and healthy.

You can serve with a side salad for dinner and top with smoked salmon and capers.

PREP TIME: 15 mins
COOK TIME: 10 mins
TOTAL TIME: 25 mins
YIELD: 1 serving

NUTRITIONAL INFO

Calories: 150 cal | **Total fat**: 9 g | **Saturated Fat:** 2 g | **Sodium:** 300 mg | **Sugar:** 2 g | **Cholesterol:** 190 mg | **Carbohydrates:** 7 g | **Protein:** 10 g | **Fiber:** 1 mg

INGREDIENTS

- 1 tablespoon of olive oil
- 1 small red onion, minced
- 1 clove garlic, minced
- 4 eggs, whisked
- 1 tablespoon of minced fresh chives
- 1 cup of (250 ml) coarsely chopped kale, stems removed
- 2 ounces of (60 grams) smoked salmon, thinly sliced
- 1 tablespoon of capers (optional)

DIRECTIONS

- Heat oil over medium-low heat in a skillet and sauté garlic with onion for about 3 minutes.
- Add chives and eggs.
- Stir and continue cooking for about 3 minutes.
- Place kale over the omelet and fold omelet in half. Continue cooking for 1 min.
- Top with capers and smoked salmon, if using.
- Serve yourself and enjoy.

BROCCOLI SALAD

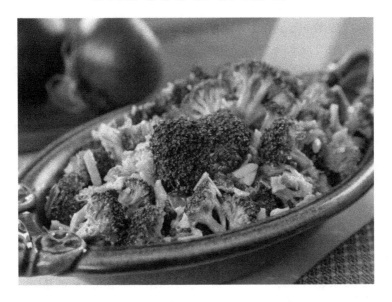

This kind of salad is a yummy breakfast salad that uses an exciting combination of vegetables, fruits, and meats. It would be best if you tried this meal before you decide you won't like it.

This recipe is packed with a wide array of vitamins, fiber, minerals, and other bio-active compounds. It has lots of advantages in its nutrient content. For this recipe, you can add an extra head of broccoli if you feel like it.

PREP TIME: 15 mins
COOK TIME: 15 mins
TOTAL TIME: 30 mins
YIELD: 1 serving

NUTRITIONAL INFO

Calories: 373.8 cal | **Total fat:** 27.2 g | **Saturated Fat:** 4.4 g | **Sodium:** 325.9 mg | **Sugar:** 20.3 g | **Vitamin B6:** 0.3mg | **Iron:** 0.9 mg | **Cholesterol:** 18.3 mg | **Carbohydrates:** 28.5 g | **Protein:** 7.3 g | **Vitamin C:** 60.7 mg | **Potassium:** 416 mg | **Calcium:** 64.4 mg

INGREDIENTS

- 1 - 1/2 teaspoon of raisins
- 1 tablespoon and 1 teaspoon of sliced almonds
- 1 tablespoon and 2-1/4 teaspoons of mayonnaise
- 2-3/4 teaspoons of white sugar
- 1/4 head of fresh broccoli
- 1/8 red onion
- 1 ounce of bacon
- 3/4 teaspoon of white wine vinegar

DIRECTIONS

- In a deep skillet, place bacon and cook over medium high heat until evenly brown. Cool and crumble.
- Cut the onion into thin bite size slices and the broccoli into bite size pieces.
- Combine with raisins, bacon, and your favorite nuts and mix well.
- To prepare the dressing, mix the sugar, mayonnaise, and vinegar together until smooth.
- Stir into the salad and let it chill.
- Serve and enjoy your meal.

APPLE CINNAMON OMELET

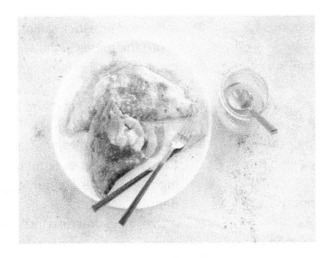

This is a delicious baked omelet using fresh apples. You can multiply the flavor by adding more apples. It's one of the best omelets you'll never forget because of its uniqueness.

This meal is loaded with antioxidants. The most exciting part of it is that it has a robust anti-diabetic effect and lowers your blood sugar. So I think this is one of the best breakfast recipes you should try!

PREP TIME: 10 mins
COOK TIME: 0 mins
TOTAL TIME: 10 mins
YIELD: 1 serving

NUTRITIONAL INFO

Calories: 379 cal | **Total fat:** 17 g | **Saturated Fat:** 9 g | **Sodium:** 525 mg | **Sugar:** 18 g | **Vitamin A:** 905iu | **Iron:** 3.9 mg | **Cholesterol:** 243 mg | **Carbohydrates:** 62 g | **Protein:** 17 g | **Vitamin C:** 1/2 mg | **Potassium:** 538 mg | **Fiber:** 1 mg | **Calcium:** 268 mg

INGREDIENTS

- 3 tablespoons of water
- 1/8 teaspoon of salt
- 1/8 teaspoon of pepper
- 1/2 cup of thinly sliced peeled tart apple
- 2 teaspoons of sugar
- 1/4 teaspoon of ground cinnamon
- 2 tablespoons of butter, divided
- 3 large eggs
- Sweetened whipped cream

DIRECTIONS

- In a small nonstick skillet, sauté the apple, sugar, cinnamon in 1 tablespoon of butter.
- Remove from skillet and set it aside.
- Melt the rest of the butter in the same skillet over medium high heat. Whisk water, eggs, pepper, and salt.
- Add the egg mixture into the skillet.
- Push cooked edges as eggs set toward the center, letting uncooked portion flow underneath.
- Spoon apple mixture on one side when the eggs are set.
- Fold other side overfilling. Slide omelet onto a plate.
- Serve with whipped cream and enjoy.

MUSHROOM KALE WITH FRITTATA

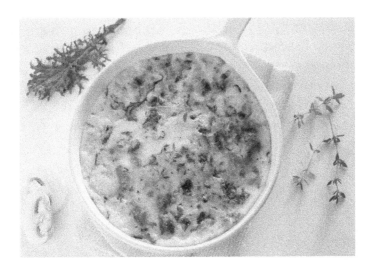

You need this recipe to protect the body from damaging free radicals that can cause conditions like cancer and heart disease.

This frittata is so quick, easy, and perfect as a quick breakfast. It is excellent when served warm or at room temperature, making it the perfect make-ahead dish.

PREP TIME: 15 mins
COOK TIME: 10 mins
TOTAL TIME: 25 mins
YIELD: 1 serving

NUTRITIONAL INFO

Calories: 269 cal | Total fat: 21 g | Saturated Fat: 5.9 g | Sodium: 450 mg | Sugar: 1 g | Iron: 2 mg | Cholesterol: 378 mg | Carbohydrates: 4 g | Protein: 16 g | Fiber: 1 g | Calcium: 147 mg

INGREDIENTS

- 2 large eggs
- 1/2 cup of sliced cremini mushrooms
- 1/2 cup of loosely packed baby kale or spinach
- 1 tablespoon of feta cheese or crumbled goat
- 1/4 teaspoon of freshly ground black pepper, divided
- 1/8 teaspoon of kosher salt, divided 2 teaspoons of olive oil

DIRECTIONS

- Preheat broiler to high and set a rack 6 inches from the heat.
- In a small bowl, break the eggs and use a fork to beat them like a bass drum until completely blended and slightly frothy.
- Stir in half of the salt and pepper.
- In an 8-inch cast-iron skillet, heat olive oil over medium high.
- Add the mushrooms to pan and saute until nicely browned.
- Stir in the remaining salt and pepper and kale as well.
- Sauté until kale is just wilted.
- Add eggs and stir slowly when the eggs are lightly browned on the bottom with a few shiny spots still on top, for about 2 minutes. Sprinkle with cheese.
- Place the pan under broiler and broil till golden brown spots appear on egg and cheese softens.
- Slide the frittata onto a plate and enjoy.

CITRUS SALAD WITH KALE

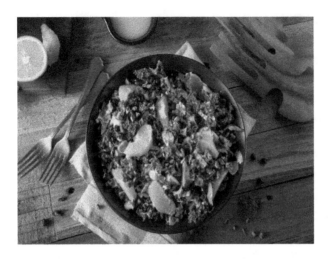

Loads of kale, red onion, green apple, pomegranate, cranberries, and grapefruit to make this Salad hearty and substantial.

This is the best if you love crisp salads with a balance of sweet and tart. Kale Citrus Salad is one of the best healthy breakfast recipes on your daily to-do list.

PREP TIME: 30 mins
COOK TIME: 0 mins
TOTAL TIME: 30 mins
YIELD: 1 serving

NUTRITIONAL INFO

Calories: 239 cal | **Total fat:** 17 g | **Saturated Fat:** 2.4 g | **Sodium:** 100 mg | **Sugar:** 11.7 g | **Iron:** 0 mg | **Cholesterol:** 0 mg | **Carbohydrates:** 21 g | **Protein:** 2.8 g | **Fiber:** 3 g | **Calcium:** 0 mg

INGREDIENTS

Pickled Onions:
- 0.06 red onion (thinly sliced)
- 0.08 cup of red wine vinegar
- 0.25 tablespoon of sugar
- 0.5 tablespoon of water

Salad:
- 0.25 large bundle lacinato kale (1 large bundle yields 4 cups, chopped)
- 0.06 cup of dried cranberries or pomegranate arils (you can use mix both)
- 0.25 grapefruit or orange (segmented or reserve any juice)
- 0.25 tart apple (chopped and cored)

Dressing:
- 0.13 tablespoon of sweetener of choice (such as maple syrup or honey, if not vegan)

DIRECTIONS

- Pickle onions by mixing water, red wine vinegar, and sugar in a small bowl, stirring to dissolve.
- Add the sliced onions and let it set in the fridge. Prep the rest of the salad while the onion is in fridge.
- The liquid should cover the onion, so add a bit more water and/or vinegar if needed.
- In a large mixing bowl with 2 teaspoons of olive oil, add kale and squeeze over reserved orange juice or grapefruit.
- Break down the stiffness and bitterness of the kale by using your fingers to massage it.
- The next thing you'll want to do is add orange segments, grapefruits, and cranberries or pomegranate and set it aside.
- In a small mixing bowl, prepare dressing by whisking mustard, vinegar, salt, sweetener, and pepper.
- Stream in olive oil while mixing, then taste and maybe, adjust seasonings.
- You can add a splash of orange juice to give more flavors.

48

- 0.08 cup of olive oil (plus more for massaging kale)
- 0.75 tablespoon of red wine vinegar
- 0.25 tablespoon of Dijon mustard
- pinch sea salt + black pepper
- 0.5 tablespoon of orange juice (to brighten the flavor) - this is optional.

Toppings (optional):

- Roasted nuts, hemp-seeds or sunflower seeds (for extra protein)
- Berries in spring and summer
- Cooked quinoa

- Add your pickled onions to the salad and dressing.
- Toss and serve.
- Enjoy.

BERRIES ARUGULA WITH SALAD

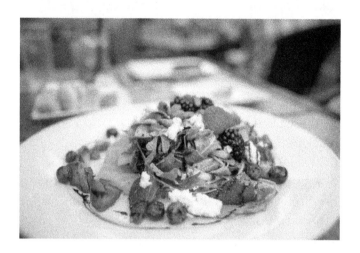

I love the word 'Arugula,' and it's perfectly okay for this recipe. It is loaded with berries like blueberries and strawberries, coupled with creamy goat cheese. It would be great if you can drizzle with the best balsamic glaze!

Berries Arugula with Salad is my to-go morning meal. You can add some fruit to this salad. This will give it a winning combination.

With just five (5) ingredients, prepare your Berries Arugula Salad and get the most excellent flavor for your breakfast. It's so fast, easy to make, and always disappears fast.

PREP TIME: 10 mins
COOK TIME: 10 mins
TOTAL TIME: 20 mins
YIELD: 1 serving

NUTRITIONAL INFO

Calories: 92 cal | **Total fat:** 21 g | **Saturated Fat:** 5.9 g | **Sodium:** 450 mg | **Sugar:** 1 g | **Iron:** 2 mg | **Cholesterol:** 378 mg | **Carbohydrates:** 4 g | **Protein:** 16 g | **Fiber:** 1 g | **Calcium:** 147 mg

INGREDIENTS

- 1 ounce of blueberries
- 0.67 ounce of goat cheese crumbled
- 0.83 ounces of baby arugula
- 1.33 ounces of strawberries sliced and hulled
- 0.33 tablespoon of balsamic glaze or added to taste

DIRECTIONS

- In a large salad bowl, place your arugula and top with sliced strawberries, crumbled goat cheese, and whole blueberries.
- Drizzle the top with balsamic glaze.
- Add it to taste and serve.
- Make sure you don't toss this salad because it serves beautifully. You just have to drizzle and leave it like that.
- Enjoy.

GRANOLA BUCKWHEAT

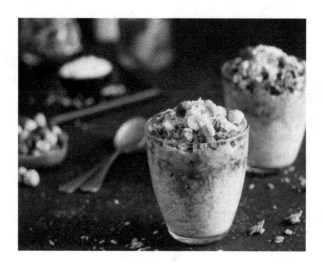

Get yourself a bowl of wholesome, tasty, and extra crunchy granola today. It's so simple! And to make it, it requires just ten (10) ingredients.

It starts with an even mixture of buckwheat groats and oats, but you can use all buckwheat groats if you feel like.

Next, come coconut and nuts, a little maple syrup and coconut sugar for natural sweetness, and a little cinnamon for warmth. I wish you could smell it through the book right now.

PREP TIME: 5 mins
COOK TIME: 25 mins
TOTAL TIME: 30 mins
YIELD: 1 serving

NUTRITIONAL INFO

Calories: 186 cal | **Total fat:** 8.7 g | **Saturated Fat:** 4 g | **Sodium:** 64 mg | **Sugar:** 8.7 g | **Iron:** 0 mg | **Cholesterol:** 0 mg | **Carbohydrates:** 25.4 g | **Protein:** 3.5 g | **Fiber:** 3.8 g | **Potassium:** 79 mg

INGREDIENTS

- 0.03 cup of unsweetened coconut flakes (or shredded coconut)
- 0.11 tablespoon of chia seeds (or flax seeds)
- 0.16 tablespoon of coconut sugar (or another dry sweetener of choice)
- 0.03 teaspoon of sea salt
- 0.04 teaspoon of ground cinnamon
- 0.08 cups of raw buckwheat groats
- 0.08 cups of gluten-free rolled oats (or sub all buckwheat groats)
- 0.04 cup of chopped raw nuts or seeds (cashews, pecans, and/or walnuts are best, or sunflower seeds or sub sesame)
- 0.01 cup of coconut, avocado, or olive oil

DIRECTIONS

- Preheat oven to 325 degrees F.
- Add the oats, buckwheat groats, nuts, chia seeds, coconut, sea salt, coconut sugar, and cinnamon into a mixing bowl. Stir to combine.
- Warm the maple syrup and oil in a small saucepan over medium-low heat until combined and melted.
- Then add the nut butter and stir again to combine.
- Pour over the dry ingredients and mix them well to coat.
- Spread the mixture evenly onto a baking sheet and bake for about 25 minutes, stirring a bit halfway point to ensure even baking.
- While the granola is still warm, add the dried fruit.
- Wait until it has cooled completely if adding chocolate.
- In a sealed container, place cooled granola that has an air-tight seal and you can store in the freezer for one month or longer.
- Enjoy.

- 0.03 cup of maple syrup (plus more to taste / or other liquid sweetener of choice)
- 0.16 tablespoon of seed butter or nut (optional - I prefer almond or peanut)
- 0.02 cup of dried fruit

For Serving (optional):
- Dairy-free milk
- Fresh fruit

APPLE CAKES

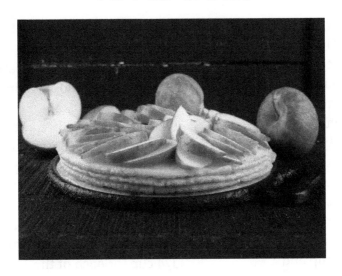

This is a delicious recipe that is perfect for your morning breakfast, and they are an ideal way to sneak some healthy fruit into your breakfast routine.

These pancakes are so nutritious and are always moist. I highly recommend these pancakes to be eaten with hot cinnamon syrup!

PREP TIME: 10 mins
COOK TIME: 20 mins
TOTAL TIME: 35 mins
YIELD: 1 serving

NUTRITIONAL INFO

Calories: 92 cal | Total fat: 21 g | Saturated Fat: 5.9 g | Sodium: 450 mg | Sugar: 1 g | Iron: 2 mg | Cholesterol: 378 mg | Carbohydrates: 4 g | Protein: 16 g | Fiber: 1 g | Calcium: 147 mg

INGREDIENTS

- 1/4 teaspoon of baking powder
- 1/8 teaspoon of ground cinnamon
- 3/4 teaspoon of white sugar
- 1 tablespoon of butter, melted
- 1/4 egg
- 1/4 cup of milk
- 1/4 cup of shredded tart apple
- 1/4 cup and 1 tablespoon of all-purpose flour

DIRECTIONS

- Combine egg, butter, apple, and milk in a large bowl.
- Sift together cinnamon, baking powder, flour, and sugar in a separate bowl.
- Stir the apple mixture into the flour mixture and just until combined.
- Heat a lightly oiled frying pan over medium high heat.
- Scoop or pour the batter onto the frying pan, using approx 1/4 cup for each of the pancakes.
- Brown on both sides.
- Serve hot and enjoy.

SALMON WITH SCRAMBLED EGG

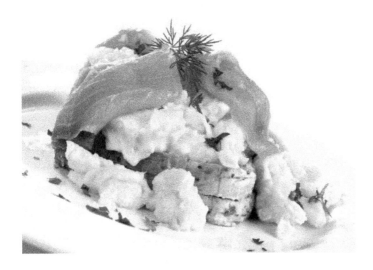

I am sure you love eggs. Now, this recipe is just the best for you. You can add some ingredients like red capsicum, trim milk, salmon, black pepper, and parsley. Wow, this would be great and delicious seriously.

You need to brighten up your day and put a smile on your face in the morning. So try this scrambled eggs with salmon and see the magic!

PREP TIME: 10 mins
COOK TIME: 10 mins
TOTAL TIME: 20 mins
YIELD: 1 serving

NUTRITIONAL INFO

Calories: 92 cal | **Total fat:** 21 g | **Saturated Fat:** 5.9 g | **Sodium:** 450 mg | **Sugar:** 1 g | **Iron:** 2 mg | **Cholesterol:** 378 mg | **Carbohydrates:** 4 g | **Protein:** 16 g | **Fiber:** 1 g | **Calcium:** 147 mg

INGREDIENTS

- 0.25 of diced red capsicum
- 2 eggs
- 3 tablespoons of trim milk
- 57 to 75g cooked salmon
- freshly ground black pepper
- 1 tablespoon of chopped fresh parsley
- 1/2 panini
- slices of lemon

DIRECTIONS

- In a small microwave-proof dish, place capsicum and cook on high for about 30 seconds.
- Set it aside. Then break salmon into bite-sized pieces.
- In a microwave-proof container, beat eggs together with milk. Heat on high for about 1 minute. Beat using fork and cook for another 1 seconds.
- Beat again and cook for another 30 seconds.
- Remove from the heat and add salmon and diced capsicum.
- Lightly mix together and cook for a final 30 seconds
- This time, the eggs should look a little wet.
- Season with parsley and pepper. Leave it to stand for 60 seconds.
- Meanwhile, heat panini for about 30 seconds and then slice.
- Place on your serving plate.
- Top with scrambled eggs.
- Serve with a slice of lemon immediately and enjoy.

SPINACH WITH EGG SCRAMBLE

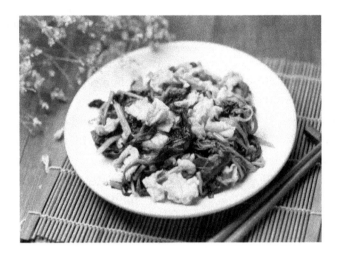

Adding spinach to your egg scramble is a great and excellent source of vitamin A, vitamin K, and vitamin C. They are essential for maintaining bone health, and it is difficult to find vegetables richer than spinach.

Enjoy spinach with egg scramble today and stay healthy!

PREP TIME: 10 mins
COOK TIME: 10 mins
TOTAL TIME: 20 mins
YIELD: 1 serving

NUTRITIONAL INFO

Calories: 303 cal | **Total fat:** 25 g | **Saturated Fat:** 6 g | **Sodium:** 612 mg | **Sugar:** 2 g | **Iron:** 0 mg | **Cholesterol:** 0 mg | **Carbohydrates:** 4 g | **Protein:** 16 g | **Fiber:** 0 g | **Calcium:** 0 mg

INGREDIENTS

- 1 tablespoon (1 ounce) of grated Parmesan
- 1 cup (2 ounces) of fresh baby spinach leaves
- 0.13 teaspoon of red pepper flakes
- 1 tablespoon of olive oil
- 0.25 of sliced medium onion, separated into rings
- 0.25 teaspoon of kosher salt with a pinch for the onions
- 0.13 teaspoon of black pepper, divided
- 2 large eggs

DIRECTIONS

- Heat a 12-inch large nonstick skillet over medium-high heat, for about 2 minutes.
- Add the olive oil and the sliced onion.
- Sprinkle them with a pinch of kosher salt and black pepper.
- Cook, stirring very well, for about 5 minutes, until golden. Lower the heat to medium.
- Whisk together 1/2 teaspoon of kosher salt, eggs, 2 tablespoons of Parmesan, and a pinch of black pepper in a medium bowl. Do this while the onion is cooking and set it aside.
- Add the spinach leaves to the skillet when the onions are golden brown.
- Cook and stir for about a minute, until it begins to wilt.
- Pour the egg mixture into the skillet, then cook the eggs over medium heat, using rubber spatula to push them back and forth, until set to your liking.
- Sprinkle with red pepper flakes.
- Serve immediately and enjoy.

VEGGIE OMELET

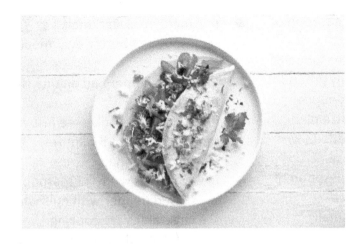

Veggie Omelet is a delicious and healthy recipe that lets you use your favorite veggie to create your perfect omelet. They are easy-to-prepare recipes and loaded with lots of vegetables to make a high protein and satisfying meal.

Enjoy this omelet served on top of toast!

PREP TIME: 10 mins
COOK TIME: 15 mins
TOTAL TIME: 25 mins
YIELD: 1 serving

NUTRITIONAL INFO

Calories: 386.4 cal | **Total fat:** 29.8 g | **Saturated Fat:** 6 g | **Sodium:** 15.7 mg | **Sugar:** 4.8 g | **Iron:** 2.2 mg | **Cholesterol:** 429.8 mg | **Carbohydrates:** 9.1 g | **Protein:** 21.7 g | **Fiber:** 0 g | **Calcium:** 313.6 mg

INGREDIENTS

- 1/4 teaspoon of salt
- 1/8 teaspoon of freshly ground black pepper
- 1 ounce of shredded Swiss cheese
- 1 tablespoon of butter
- 1/2 small chopped onion
- 1/2 green chopped bell pepper
- 2 eggs
- 1 tablespoon of milk

DIRECTIONS

- In a medium skillet, melt 1 tablespoon of butter over medium heat.
- Place bell pepper and onion inside the skillet.
- Cook until vegetables are just tender, for about 5 minutes, stirring occasionally.
- Beat the eggs with 1/2 teaspoon of salt and pepper with milk while the vegetables are cooking.
- In a small bowl, shred the cheese and set it aside.
- Remove the vegetables from the heat.
- Transfer them into a separate bowl and sprinkle the rest of the salt over them.
- Melt the rest of the butter over medium heat.
- Coat the skillet with the butter.
- Add the egg mixture while the butter is bubbly and cook the egg until the eggs begin to set on the bottom of the pan, for about 2 minutes.
- Lift the edges of the omelet gently using a spatula to let the uncooked part of the eggs flows to the edges and cook.
- Continue cooking until the center of the omelet starts to look dry, for about 3 minutes.

- Sprinkle the cheese over the omelet.
- Spoon the vegetable mixture into the center of the omelet.
- Over the vegetables, using a spatula to gently fold one edge of the omelet.
- Let the omelet cook until the cheese melts to your desired consistency, for about 2 minutes.
- Slide the omelet out of the skillet and place on a plate.
- Cut into half, serve and enjoy.

COCONUT PORRIDGE

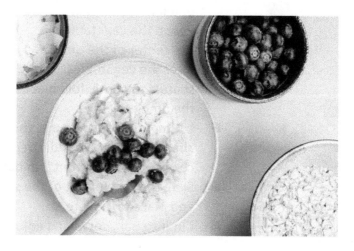

It would be best if you combined until you achieve a thick, creamy texture for this coconut porridge. This recipe is a simple warming coconut flour porridge for a quiet morning.

It's a low-carb and keto breakfast option as well. You can enjoy a warm and nutritious bowl of this oats for breakfast when you're craving for it.

PREP TIME: 10 mins
COOK TIME: 10 mins
TOTAL TIME: 20 mins
YIELD: 1 serving

NUTRITIONAL INFO

Calories: 487 cal | **Total fat:** 39.3 g | **Saturated Fat:** 89% g | **Sodium:** 357 mg | **Sugar:** 3 g | **Iron:** 1 mg | **Cholesterol:** 61 mg | **Carbohydrates:** 11.3 g | **Protein:** 9 g | **Fiber:** 6.3 g | **Calcium:** 17 mg

INGREDIENTS

- 1 ounce of coconut oil or butter
- 4 tablespoons of coconut cream
- 1 beaten egg
- 1 pinch of salt
- 1 tablespoon of coconut flour
- 1 pinch of ground psyllium husk powder

DIRECTIONS

- Combine the coconut flour, egg, psyllium husk powder, and salt in a small bowl.
- Melt the butter and coconut cream over low heat.
- Whisk in the egg mixture slowly, combining until you achieve a thick creamy texture.
- Serve with cream or coconut milk.
- Top your porridge with some fresh or frozen berries.
- Serve and enjoy.

SWISS CARD WITH CHICKPEA

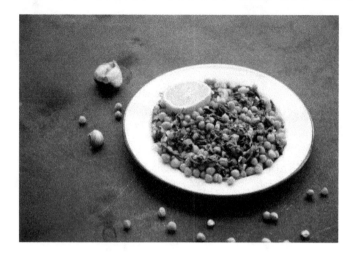

This recipe is as fresh as morning. Spinach is an authentic substitute if you can't find Swiss Chard.

PREP TIME: 20 mins
COOK TIME: 0 mins
TOTAL TIME: 20 mins
YIELD: 1 serving

NUTRITIONAL INFO

Calories: 303 cal | **Total fat:** 25 g | **Saturated Fat:** 6 g | **Sodium:** 612 mg | **Sugar:** 2 g | **Iron:** 0 mg | **Cholesterol:** 0 mg | **Carbohydrates:** 4 g | **Protein:** 16 g | **Fiber:** 0 g | **Calcium:** 0 mg

INGREDIENTS

- 1/2 cup of rinsed canned chickpeas
- 0.25 pound of Swiss chard, stems discarded and leaves coarsely chopped
- 0.25 tablespoon of fresh lemon juice
- 1/2 small onion (thinly sliced)
- 1/2 garlic clove (thinly sliced)
- 1 tablespoon of olive oil
- 1/2 small tomato, cut into 1/4-inch dice

DIRECTIONS

- In a large nonstick skillet, cook onion and garlic over medium low heat.
- Stir until softened.
- Add chickpeas and tomato.
- Cook, stirring, for about 5 minutes.
- Add your Swiss chard and cook.
- Cover it for about 2 minutes, until wilted.
- Add lemon juice.
- Season with pepper and salt.
- Enjoy.

PAK CHOI STIR FRY WITH PRAWNS

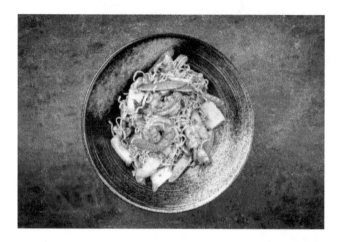

Within 11 minutes, your prawn stir-fry can be thrown together and served. The combination of Pak-Choi and prawns makes a perfect morning.

This meal is highly nutritious and packed with vitamins, fiber, minerals, and some antioxidants.

PREP TIME: 5 mins
COOK TIME: 6 mins
TOTAL TIME: 11 mins
YIELD: 1 serving

NUTRITIONAL INFO

Calories: 484 cal | **Total fat:** 20 g | **Saturated Fat:** 3 g | **Sodium:** 0 mg | **Sugar:** 9 g | **Iron:** 0 mg | **Cholesterol:** 0 mg | **Carbohydrates:** 48 g | **Protein:** 25 g | **Fiber:** 7 g | **Calcium:** 0 mg

INGREDIENTS

- 1 spring onion, sliced on the diagonal
- 150grams of straight-to-wok egg noodles
- 75grams of cooked king prawns
- 1 tablespoon of sesame oil
- 50grams of mange tout
- 1/2 finely sliced carrot
- 100grams of pak choi, sliced and washed
- 1 tablespoon of soy sauce, plus extra to serve, (optional)
- 1/2 tablespoon of sesame seeds, toasted
- 1/2 red chili, sliced, to serve (optional)

DIRECTIONS

- In a large frying pan, heat 1/2 tablespoon of sesame oil over medium-high heat.
- Toss in carrot and mangetout.
- Cook until starting to brown and soften, then add the spring onion and Pak-Choi.
- Add the prawns and noodles, using your tongs to combine together, and warm through.
- Pour in the soy sauce and the rest of the sesame oil and toss to coat. Do this just before serving.
- Scatter over the chili and sesame seeds.
- Serve with extra soy sauce if you feel like.
- Enjoy.

ARUGULA SALAD WITH NUTS

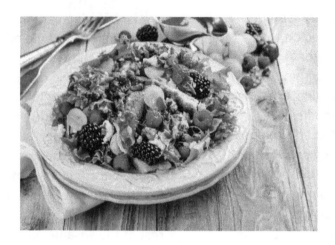

Arugula salad is made with strawberries, red onion, feta cheese, toasted pecans, and baby arugula. It's so perfect for breakfast with its fresh and light flavors.

Arugula is one of the brassica family vegetables, cabbage, cauliflower, and broccoli, that helps in detoxifying and cleansing the body.

PREP TIME: 10 mins
COOK TIME: 0 mins
TOTAL TIME: 10 mins
YIELD: 1 serving

NUTRITIONAL INFO

Calories: 144 cal | **Total fat:** 13 g | **Saturated Fat:** 2 g | **Sodium:** 76 mg | **Sugar:** 4 g | **Iron:** 0 mg | **Cholesterol:** 6 mg | **Carbohydrates:** 5 g | **Protein:** 2 g | **Fiber:** 1 g | **Calcium:** 69 mg

INGREDIENTS

Salad
- 1/2 cup of feta cheese crumbled
- 1/2 cup of red onion sliced
- 1 tablespoon of toasted walnuts or pecans
- 3 cups of baby arugula
- 1/2 cup of cherries pitted
- 1/2 cup of strawberries or blackberries/raspberries

Dressing
- 1 1/2 tablespoons of olive oil or vegetable oil
- 1 teaspoon of honey
- 1 tablespoon of rice vinegar
- Pepper and salt to taste

DIRECTIONS

- Add together the berries, arugula, red onion, feta cheese and nuts in a medium bowl.
- In a mason jar, combine all of the dressing ingredients and shake well.
- Pour over the salad.
- Toss and serve.
- Enjoy.

SWEET POTATO FRIES WITH AVOCADO DIP

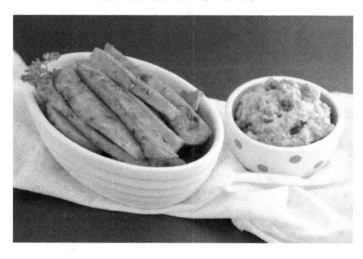

Do you know that this recipe is so soft on the inside and crispy on the outside?

These sweet potato fries with avocado dip make a perfect healthy breakfast meal. They are super quick and easy to prepare. You can have this dish when watching a movie. I bet you. There is absolutely no reason not to try this recipe!

PREP TIME: 10 mins
COOK TIME: 25 mins
TOTAL TIME: 35 mins
YIELD: 1 serving

NUTRITIONAL INFO

Calories: 428 cal | **Total fat:** 35.4 g | **Saturated Fat:** 7.5 g | **Sodium:** 96 mg | **Sugar:** 9.9 g | **Iron:** 1 mg | **Cholesterol:** 7 mg | **Carbohydrates:** 20.2 g | **Protein:** 9.6 g | **Fiber:** 7.4 g | **Calcium:** 246 mg

INGREDIENTS

Sweet Potato Fries:
- 1/2 teaspoon of paprika
- 1/2 teaspoon of garlic powder
- Black pepper and salt
- 1 large sweet potatoes, cut into sticks
- 1 tablespoon of olive oil

Avocado Dip:
- 1/2 cup (60 ml) of plain yogurt
- 1 tablespoon of fresh lemon juice
- 1 garlic cloves, crushed
- 1/2 ripe avocado
- Pepper and salt
- Fresh cilantro, cut

DIRECTIONS

- Preheat the oven to 400 degrees F.
- Use parchment paper to line a baking tray
- Cut the sweet potatoes into sticks, about 1/2 inch wide.
- Use olive oil to toss them in a large mixing bowl.
- Add the garlic, paprika, pepper, and salt and toss well.
- Transfer the sweet potatoes into the prepared baking sheet.
- Bake until crisp and brown on the bottom, for about 10 to 15 minutes, then flip.
- Bake for about 10 minutes, until the other side is crisp.
- Prepare the avocado dip in the meantime: Mix the garlic cloves until minced in a food processor.
- Add the yogurt, ripe avocado, fresh lemon juice and mix until smooth texture.
- Season with pepper and salt.
- Add cilantro on top
- Serve and enjoy.

SALMON WITH CAPERS

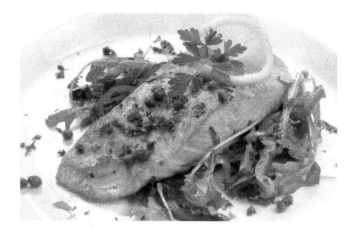

This kind of recipe is an easy pan-seared salmon recipe that is ready in a flash and allows the salmon's flavor to smell nice.

This is a delicious sauce of lemon, butter, and capers that can be put together and ready within 15 minutes. Eating this recipe in the morning will help protect your heart.

PREP TIME: 5 mins
COOK TIME: 10 mins
TOTAL TIME: 15 mins
YIELD: 1 serving

NUTRITIONAL INFO

Calories: 354 cal | **Total fat:** 23 g | **Saturated Fat:** 6 g | **Sodium:** 241 mg | **Sugar:** 0 g | **Iron:** 0 mg | **Cholesterol:** 108 mg | **Carbohydrates:** 0 g | **Protein:** 33 g | **Fiber:** 0 g | **Calcium:** 20 mg

INGREDIENTS

- 1 6-ounces of salmon steaks
- 0.5 tablespoon of unsalted butter
- 1 Lemon juice
- 0.75 tablespoon of capers
- 0.5 tablespoon of olive oil
- lemon slices for garnishing

DIRECTIONS

- Heat a heavy skillet over medium heat until hot, for about 2 minutes.
- Increase heat to medium-high and then add olive oil.
- Place the salmon steaks flesh side down in the pan when the surface of the oil starts shimmering.
- Cook for about 3 minutes.
- Turn the salmon over and cook until the fish is flaky and opaque in color, for about additional 5 minutes.
- Remove from pan and place over a serving platter.
- Reduce the heat to medium, add the lemon juice, add the butter, and capers to the pan.
- Then cook, stirring constantly, until the sauce has combined and butter has melted.
- Drizzle the sauce over the salmon.
- Garnish with lemon slices.
- Serve immediately and enjoy.

Lunch
Recipes

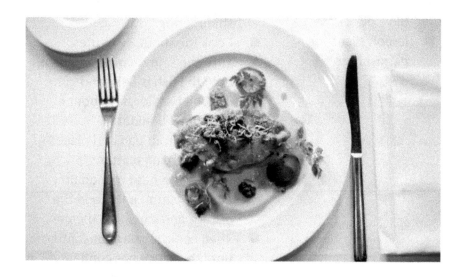

Adele Bayles

MEDITERRANEAN PIZZA

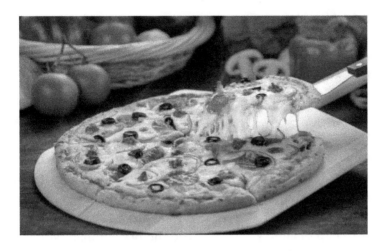

This is a delicious pizza recipe. It's packed with different Mediterranean toppings.

You're going to love this pizza with marinated artichokes, fresh tomatoes, and delicious veggies. I'm confident this pizza is going to be your new favorite lunch meal.

You would love it!

PREP TIME: 15 mins
COOK TIME: 15 mins
TOTAL TIME: 30 mins
YIELD: 1 serving

NUTRITIONAL INFO

Calories: 507 cal | **Total fat:** 21.3 g | **Saturated Fat:** 2.7 g | **Sodium:** 1084 mg | **Sugar:** 0 g | **Iron:** 0 mg | **Cholesterol:** 4 mg | **Carbohydrates:** 74.3 g | **Protein:** 13.8 g | **Fiber:** 6.8 g | **Calcium:** 34 mg

INGREDIENTS

- 0.25 12-inch pizza dough (store-bought or homemade)
- 0.25 teaspoon of thyme
- 0.19 cup of red onion sliced
- 0.25 cup of fresh mozzarella, shredded or sliced
- 0.13 cup of cherry tomatoes halved
- 0.13 cup of fresh parsley chopped
- 0.06 teaspoon of black pepper
- 0.13 teaspoon of dried basil optional
- 0.25 (15 ounces) can of artichoke hearts
- 1 tablespoon of olive oil extra virgin
- 0.13 teaspoon of salt
- 0.19 cup of sun-dried tomatoes
- 0.13 cup of Kalamata olive, halved and pitted

DIRECTIONS

- Preheat the oven to 375 degrees F.
- Place it in the oven if you're using a pizza stone.
- Roll out the pizza dough to 12 inches on a pizza peel or baking sheet.
- Spread the olive oil on the dough, then sprinkle salt, black pepper, thyme, and dried basil on the pizza dough.
- Top the pizza dough with sun dried tomatoes, artichoke hearts, red onion, olives, and fresh mozzarella.
- Transfer the pizza onto the pizza stone if you'll be using it.
- Bake in the oven until cheese is bubbly and melted, for about 15 minutes.
- Top with chopped parsley and fresh tomatoes.
- Serve immediately and enjoy.

SHRIMP SKILLET WITH KALE

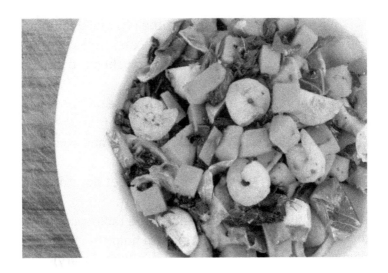

This recipe only requires four (4) ingredients, gluten-free, and super easy to make. It only takes a few minutes to be ready and place on your table. But the sweet potatoes take a little time to cook.

PREP TIME: 5 mins
COOK TIME: 15 mins
TOTAL TIME: 25 mins
YIELD: 1 serving

NUTRITIONAL INFO

Calories: 265 cal | **Total fat:** 7.8g | **Sodium:** 0 mg | **Sugar:** 0 g | **Iron:** 0 mg | **Cholesterol:** 239.5 mg | **Carbohydrates:** 18 g | **Protein:** 32.1 g

INGREDIENTS

- 0.5 cups of shrimp — deveined, peeled, and thawed if frozen
- 0.75 cups of coarsely and trimmed chopped kale leaves
- salt and ground black pepper
- 0.5 tablespoons of ghee or extra virgin olive oil
- 0.13 cup of onions — diced
- pinch crushed red pepper — to taste
- 0.5 cloves garlic — minced
- 0.5 cups of sweet potatoes — diced

DIRECTIONS

- Heat the olive oil over medium heat in a cast-iron skillet.
- Add the crushed red pepper and onions.
- Cook until the onions are golden and soft.
- Add the garlic and cook for 30 seconds.
- Add the sweet potatoes and cook till soft.
- Add a little tablespoon of water to help steam the sweet potatoes (if necessary)
- Add the shrimp and cook until they turn pink, for about 2 minutes.
- Turn the heat to low.
- Add the kale and stir until wilted.
- Season to taste with pepper and salt.
- Serve and enjoy.

KALE SALAD WITH GINGER AND CARROT

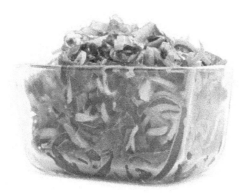

This is the kind of recipe you can combine what you have on hand to make something healthy and fresh. This salad happens when your fridge is almost empty. It's oil-free, refreshing, easy to make, and tasty. It's also perfect for a light lunch or an appetizer.

This requires just six (6) ingredients to make. So simple!

PREP TIME: 10 mins
COOK TIME: 0mins
TOTAL TIME: 10 mins
YIELD: 1 serving

NUTRITIONAL INFO

Calories: 95 cal | **Total fat:** 0 g | **Sugar:** 8.6 g | **Iron:** 0 mg | **Cholesterol:** 4 mg | **Carbohydrates:** 21.6 g | **Protein:** 3.6 g | **Fiber:** 2.6 g

INGREDIENTS

- 1 tablespoon of (15ml) of soy sauce
- 1 tablespoon of (15ml) of maple syrup
- 2 teaspoons of grated ginger
- 3 cups (180grams) of lightly packed kale
- 2 cups (100grams) of grated carrots
- 2 tablespoons (30ml) of lime juice (or white vinegar)
- for toppings, you can use roasted cashews and/or fried onions

DIRECTIONS

- Chop the kale roughly
- Add into a large mixing bowl.
- Add a pinch of salt and massage the kale until it becomes tender and turns darker, for about 1 minute.
- In a bowl, add the grated carrots and stir to mix.
- whisk together the soy sauce, lime juice, grated ginger, and maple syrup in a small bowl.
- Pour in the dressing inside the bowl, then stir to coat.
- Serve immediately
- Top with Shallots, fried onions, and/or roasted cashews.
- Enjoy.

SALMON BURGER WITH SPICY SAUCE

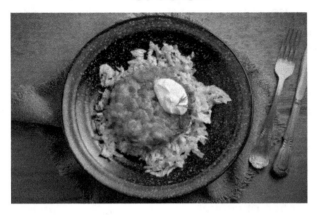

These flaky salmon burgers are filled with flavor and so rich in heart-healthy omega-3 fatty acids. It's the kind of recipe that can be jazzed up with zesty slaw and some spicy sauce or maybe, just try them plain.

This might be your first time trying it, but I promise you would fall in love. Be sure to keep some cans of salmon in your pantry. In case you might need to come up with something delicious for your lunch.

PREP TIME: 20 mins
COOK TIME: 5 mins
TOTAL TIME: 25 mins
YIELD: 1 burger

NUTRITIONAL INFO

Calories: 310 cal | **Total fat:** 17 g | **Saturated Fat:** 3 g | **Sodium:** 960 mg | **Sugar:** 0 g | **Iron:** 0 mg | **Cholesterol:** 0 mg | **Carbohydrates:** 14 g | **Protein:** 26 g | **Fiber:** 0 g | **Calcium:** 34 mg

INGREDIENTS

- 1 tablespoon of mayonnaise, lite
- 1/2 teaspoon of minced garlic
- 1/2 teaspoon of salt
- 1/2 cup of lite mayonnaise (for the slaw)
- 1/9 teaspoon of salt (for the slaw)
- 1/4 teaspoon of pepper (for the slaw)
- 1/2 teaspoon of pepper
- 1/2 3 ounces pouched or canned salmon
- 1/2 cup of panko bread crumbs
- 1/2 tablespoon of diced onion
- 1/2 teaspoon of lime juice
- 1 tablespoon of chopped cilantro
- 1 teaspoon of olive oil (for pan-searing)
- 1 tablespoon of sour cream, light (for spicy sauce)
- 1 drop of Habanero Sauce (for spicy sauce)
- 2 cups of shredded cabbage (for the slaw)
- 1/2 cup of shredded

DIRECTIONS

- Combine the bread crumbs, canned salmon, lime juice, mayonnaise, onion, garlic, and cilantro in a bowl.
- Stir until it's well combined.
- Combine this mixture into 2 patties.
- In a skillet, warm olive oil and heat over medium-high heat for 5 minutes on each side.
- Spicy sauce: Combine plain Greek yogurt, sour cream, and habanero sauce.
- **Making the Creamy Slaw:**
- Combine the carrots, shredded cabbage, pepper, salt, and mayonnaise in a bowl, then store in the refrigerator for at least 1/2 hour.
- Serve salmon patties on a bed of creamy slaw
- Top with 1 tablespoon of cilantro and spicy sauce.
- Enjoy.

CREAMY KALE SALAD WITH RASPBERRY

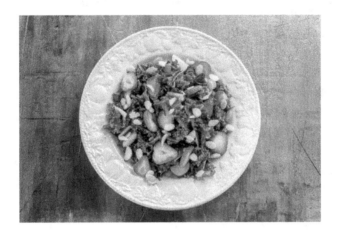

These flaky salmon burgers are filled with flavor and so rich in heart-healthy omega-3 fatty acids. It's the kind of recipe that can be jazzed up with zesty slaw and some spicy sauce or maybe, just try them plain.

This might be your first time trying it, but I promise you would fall in love. Be sure to keep some cans of salmon in your pantry. In case you might need to come up with something delicious for your lunch.

PREP TIME: 15 mins
COOK TIME:15 mins
TOTAL TIME: 25 mins
YIELD: 1 salad

NUTRITIONAL INFO

Calories: 310 cal | **Total fat:** 17 g | **Saturated Fat:** 3 g | **Sodium:** 960 mg | **Sugar:** 0 g | **Iron:** 0 mg | **Cholesterol:** 0 mg | **Carbohydrates:** 14 g | **Protein:** 26 g | **Fiber:** 0 g | **Calcium:** 34 mg

INGREDIENTS

For the salad:
- 1/2 cup of chopped green onions
- 3 tablespoons of sunflower seeds
- 1 cup of fresh raspberries (to top)
- 2 heads of Lacinato kale (about 10 cups), roughly chopped and destemmed
- 3/4 teaspoon of coarse sea salt
- 1/2 head red cabbage (about 4 cups), thinly chopped
- 1 cup of shredded carrots
- 2 tablespoons of garlic oil
- 1/2 cup of feta cheese, crumbled (to top – omit for Paleo)

For the dressing:
- 2 tablespoons of Dijon mustard
- 1 tablespoon of raw honey
- 5 tablespoons of mayo (may sub for a plain yogurt - thick)
- 2 tablespoons of red wine vinegar

DIRECTIONS

For the Salad:
- In a large bowl, add kale, garlic, and salt.
- Massage using your hand for 2 minutes.
- The kale should shrink in volume substantially and then start to tenderize.
- Add carrots, red cabbage, sunflower seeds, and green onions.
- Toss to combine.
- Reserve the feta and raspberries to top the salad after you have added the dressing.

Now let's make the dressing:
- In a medium bowl, add mayonnaise, Dijon mustard, red wine vinegar, and raw honey.
- Whisk until fully combined.
- Pour the dressing over the salad, then toss to combine.
- Add the reserved feta and raspberries to the top of the salad.
- Lightly toss.
- Serve and enjoy.

BACON WITH SWEET POTATO SALAD

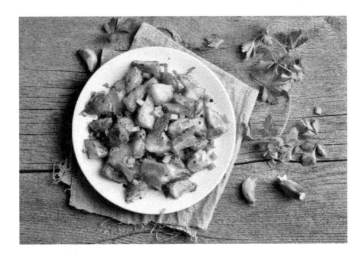

The secret of the success of this potato salad is Bacon. It adds a crisp texture and adds a smoky flavor that pairs up with the sweet potatoes nicely.

It's packed with ingredients we can easily pick from the kitchen. It's so colorful, and it's the ideal addition to your summer spread. I'm not sure you've had this kind of potato salad with Bacon. So lovely!

PREP TIME: 25 mins
COOK TIME: 2 hours
TOTAL TIME: 2 hours 25 mins
YIELD: 1 serving

NUTRITIONAL INFO

Calories: 210 cal | Total fat: 15 g | Sugar: 5 g | Iron: 4% | Cholesterol: 10 mg | Carbohydrates: 17 g | Protein: 3 g | Fiber: 3 g | Calcium: 4% | Sodium: 250 mg

INGREDIENTS

- 3/4 slices of bacon, cooked, chopped
- 1/4 cup of Mayonnaise
- 1/4 tablespoon of lime juice
- 1/4 pound of sweet potatoes, peeled, cut into 1/2-inch cubes
- 1/4 cup of chopped red pepper
- 1/4 cup of chopped celery
- 3/4 chopped green onions

DIRECTIONS

- In a large saucepan, cook potatoes in boiling water until tender, for about 10 minutes.
- Drain and rinse immediately under cold water.
- Drain and cool in a large bowl.
- Add celery, peppers, bacon, and onions to the potatoes. Toss lightly.
- Mix juice and mayonnaise until well blended.
- Pour over potato mixture.
- Stir gently and refrigerate for about 2 hours before serving.
- Serve and enjoy.

LETTUCE WRAPS

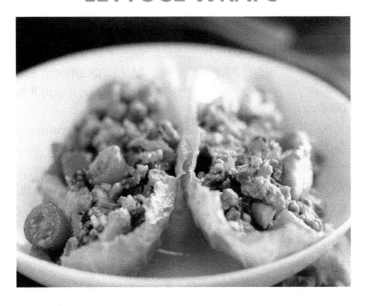

This Lettuce Wraps recipe is loaded with vegetables that are crunchy in a sweet, savory brown sauce. You can wrap with grounded shrimp or chicken.

You'll be wowed if you give this recipe a try. Lettuce wraps are so healthy, refreshing, crunchy, and delicious. They make the best light supper and taste way better than any lettuce wraps you have in mind. I'm sure of it!

PREP TIME: 20 mins
COOK TIME: 10 mins
TOTAL TIME: 30 mins
YIELD: 1 serving

NUTRITIONAL INFO

Calories: 114 cal | **Total fat:** 5 g | **Sugar:** 1 g | **Iron:** 1.2mg | **Cholesterol:** 95 mg | **Carbohydrates:** 3 g | **Protein:** 11 g | **Fiber:** 0 g | **Calcium:** 57mg | **Sodium:** 392 mg

INGREDIENTS

- Avocado oil
- 0.08 cup of chopped carrots (1 medium size carrot)
- 0.08 cup of chopped celery
- 0.5-0.63 whole water chestnuts, chopped
- 0.25 tablespoon of chopped garlic
- 0.13 large shallot, chopped
- 0.19 tablespoon of chopped ginger (3 thin slices)
- 0.06 pound of ground chicken breast
- 0.03 teaspoon of coarse salt
- 0.02 teaspoon of white pepper
- 0.06 pound of raw shrimp, diced and peeled with 1 teaspoon of arrowroot powder

Sauce (use 1 tablespoon at a time):
- 0.13 to 0.19 teaspoon of hot pepper sauce, optional
- 0.25 tablespoon of coconut Aminos

DIRECTIONS

- Get your ingredients ready and set it aside.
- Mix your shrimp with arrowroot if you'll be using.
- Add 3 tablespoons of oil in a well-heated large skillet.
- Sauté garlic, shallot, and ginger with a pinch of salt for about 10 seconds until fragrant.
- Add your ground chicken.
- Season with white pepper and salt.
- Break up the meat into fine pieces. Sauté the meal for about 5 minutes until is cooked through. This time, your skillet should not be wet or watery.
- Add celery and carrots.
- Season with a pinch of salt and sauté for about 1 minute.
- Add shrimp and chestnuts.
- Sauté for another 1 minute if you'll be using.
- Add stir-fry and sauce for 10 seconds.

- 0.06 tablespoon of almond butter
Serve and garnish:
- 0.13 whole large iceberg lettuce, leaves separated and tip edge trimmed (or 2 Boston lettuce)
- 0.38 tablespoon of lightly toasted pine nuts or chopped cashew nuts
- 0.13 bulb scallion, chopped

- Taste and make seasoning adjustments to your liking.
- Turn off the heat and garnish with scallions and pine nuts.
- Fill the lettuce cups with stir-fried ingredients.
- Serve hot and enjoy.

BRUNOISE SALAD

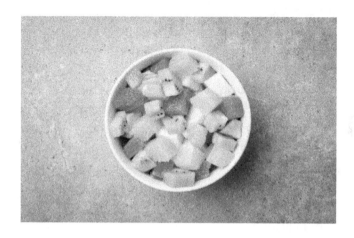

This is a delicious homemade recipe that easy to prepare and can be ready on the table within 15 minutes.

Brunoise Salad can as well be prepared for lunch, dinner, as a side dish or appetizer. This is so interesting, right?

PREP TIME: 15 mins
COOK TIME: 1 min
TOTAL TIME: 16 mins
YIELD: 1 serving

NUTRITIONAL INFO

Calories: 383 cal | **Total fat:** 28 g | **Sugar:** 0 g | **Iron:** 0mg | **Cholesterol:** 0 mg | **Carbohydrates:** 27 g | **Protein:** 6 g | **Fiber:** 8 g | **Calcium:** 0 mg | **Sodium:** 0 mg

INGREDIENTS

- 1 piece of beef tomato
- 1/2 piece of zucchini
- 1/2 piece of sweet red pepper
- 1/2 piece of yellow bell pepper
- 1/2 piece of red onion
- 3 twigs of fresh parsley
- 1/4 piece of lemon
- 2 tablespoons of olive oil
- Black pepper and salt to taste.

DIRECTIONS

- Finely dice the zucchini, tomatoes, bell peppers, and red onion, to make a brunoise.
- Mix all of the cubes in a bowl.
- Chop the parsley and mix it through the salad.
- Squeeze the lemon over the salad
- Add the olive oil.
- Season with pepper and salt.
- Serve and enjoy.

MELON SALAD WITH HAM

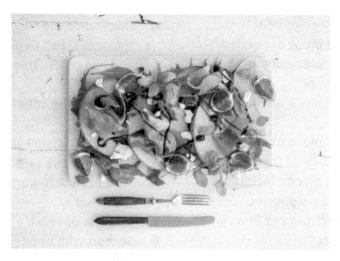

I love salads so much. This kind of salad can be prepared for breakfast, lunch, and a side dish as well.

Do you know that this recipe can help boost healthy eyesight, increase blood flow to immunity, regulate blood pressure, and be extremely robust in addition to your diet?

This is the reason you need to try it out for your lunch. So nutritious.

PREP TIME: 15 mins
COOK TIME: 0 min
TOTAL TIME: 15 mins
YIELD: 1 serving

NUTRITIONAL INFO

Calories: 476 cal | **Total fat:** 27 g | **Sugar:** 0 g | **Iron:** 0mg | **Cholesterol:** 0 mg | **Carbohydrates:** 35 g | **Protein:** 24 g | **Fiber:** 6 g | **Calcium:** 0 mg | **Sodium:** 0 mg

INGREDIENTS

- 1/2 piece of cantaloupe melon
- 4 slices of serrano ham, minced
- 100 g of arugula
- 1/2 piece of cucumber, sliced
- 1/2 piece of red onion, rings
- 1 1/2 tablespoons of olive oil

DIRECTIONS

- Cut the melon into quarters.
- Use a spoon to remove the seeds.
- Cut the skin loose and cut the melon into equal parts.
- Wrap the melon parts in ham.
- In a bowl, mix the arugula together with onion and cucumber.
- Drizzle olive oil over the salad.
- Place the wrapped melon parts on top.
- Serve and enjoy.

CAULIFLOWER PIZZA

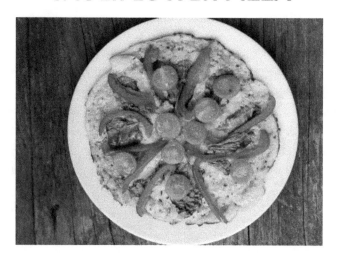

What I love about this Cauliflower Pizza are the flavors. The Meyer lemon, sun-dried tomato, and olive topping add a sophisticated Mediterranean flavor to your cauliflower pizza. Well, you can feel free to try more traditional pizza toppings.

It's mixed with oregano and mozzarella, which makes a flourless crust that echoes the flavor.

PREP TIME: 15 mins
COOK TIME: 15 min
TOTAL TIME: 30 mins
YIELD: 4 servings

NUTRITIONAL INFO

Calories: 200 cal | **Total fat:** 13.9 g | **Sugar:** 3 g | **Iron:** 1 mg | **Cholesterol:** 65 mg | **Carbohydrates:** 10.2 g | **Protein:** 10.8 g | **Fiber:** 3.2 g | **Calcium:** 256 mg | **Sodium:** 484 mg

INGREDIENTS

- 1 cup of shredded part-skim mozzarella cheese
- 1/2 teaspoon of dried oregano
- Freshly ground pepper to taste
- 1/4 cup of slivered fresh basil
- 1 medium head cauliflower (about 2 pounds), trimmed and broken into small florets
- 6 oil-packed of sun-dried tomatoes, drained and coarsely chopped
- 1/8 cup of black or green olives, pitted and sliced
- 1 large egg, lightly beaten
- 1 tablespoon plus 1 teaspoon of extra-virgin olive oil, divided
- 1/4 teaspoon of salt
- 2 Meyer lemons or 1 large regular lemon

DIRECTIONS

- Preheat the oven to 450 degrees F.
- Use parchment paper to line a pizza pan or baking sheet.
- In a food processor, place cauliflower until reduced to rice size crumbles.
- Transfer into a large nonstick skillet and add salt with 1 tablespoon of oil.
- Heat over medium-high heat, stirring frequently, for about 8 minutes, until the cauliflower starts to soften slightly.
- Transfer into a large bowl to cool for about 10 minutes.
- Remove the skin and white pith from the lemon using a sharp knife. Then discard.
- Cut the segments from the membranne in a small bowl, letting the segments to drop inside the bowl - remove seeds.
- Drain the juice from the segments.
- Add olives and tomatoes to the lemon segments.
- Toss to combine, serve, and enjoy.

ROASTED PUMPKIN SALAD

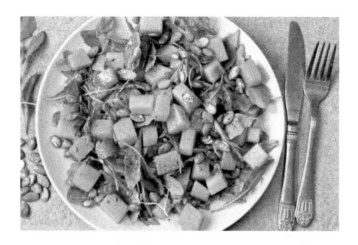

This roasted pumpkin salad is from Morocco. An aromatic Moroccan spices with hearty roast pumpkin salad - what a perfect match! This is substantial enough to energize and keep you satisfied for hours.

This is a great salad to serve with some warming casseroles or stews.

You can try it with chunky beef stew, lamb tagine, and a pork belly roast.

PREP TIME: 15 mins
COOK TIME: 30 min
TOTAL TIME: 35 mins
YIELD: 1 serving

NUTRITIONAL INFO

Calories: 311 cal | Total fat: 23 g | Sugar: 5 g | Iron: 3 mg | Cholesterol: 0 mg | Carbohydrates: 25 g | Protein: 5 g | Fiber: 5 g | Calcium: 188 mg | Sodium: 222 mg

INGREDIENTS

For roasting:
- 0.5 teaspoon of sesame oil
- 0.5-0.75 teaspoon of Ras el Hanout (depends on how much spice you like)
- Sea salt & cracked black pepper
- 0.25 butternut pumpkin (just under 1kg)
- 0.75 tablespoon of olive oil

For the salad:
- 0.5 tablespoon of sesame seeds (toasted)
- 25 grams rocket (arugula)
- 0.5 tablespoon of pepitas (toasted)

For the dressing:
- 0.25 tablespoon of soy sauce (low salt)
- 0.25 tablespoon of olive oil (extra virgin)
- 0.13 tablespoon of sesame oil
- 0.13 teaspoon of Ras el Hanout

DIRECTIONS

For the Roasting:
- Preheat oven to 180 degrees C.
- Line a baking sheet with baking paper.
- Peel the pumpkin and remove the seeds, then cut into 2.5cm pieces, placing them in a colander.
- Wash them under cold running water and drain well.
- Place the pumpkin on the tray.
- Add Ras el hanout and oils, then mix well until the pumpkin is well coated with the spice, oils and season with pepper and salt.
- Spread the pumpkin out evenly on a prepared baking sheet. Make sure the pieces don't touch so they won't turn brown and add a little water.
- In the middle section of your oven, place your baking tray and roast until golden brown and soft.
- Allow it to cool once it is done.

For the Salad:

- Wash your rocket well and remove excess water by spinning with a salad spinner. Transfer to a mixing bowl.
- In a glass jar, place all of the dressing ingredients and shake until emulsified.
- Add the cooled pumpkin into your rocket.
- Add sesame seeds and pepitas.
- Pour dressing over your salad, toss until well combined.
- Taste and adjust the seasonings according to your taste.
- In a salad bowl, arrange and scatter the reserved sesame seeds, pepitas, and the pumpkin seeds on top.
- Serve and enjoy.

CHICKEN ROLLS

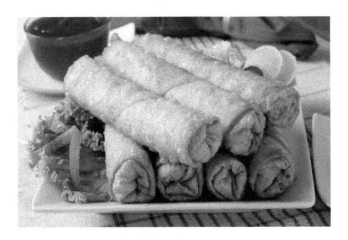

This Chicken Roll is a straightforward yet exciting dish for you and your family. It's different from your average chicken recipe.

It has a very high protein content, which plays a very vital role in sustaining our muscles.

PREP TIME: 20 mins
COOK TIME: 45 min
TOTAL TIME: 65 mins
YIELD: 4 servings

NUTRITIONAL INFO

Calories: 585.3 cal | **Total fat:** 40.3 g | **Sugar:** 0.6 g | **Iron:** 3.1 mg | **Cholesterol:** 123.5 mg | **Carbohydrates:** 5.6 g | **Protein:** 49.5 g | **Fiber:** 1.8 g | **Calcium:** 896.6 mg | **Sodium:** 886.1 mg

INGREDIENTS

- 1 skinless boneless chicken breast, halves (pounded to 1/4 inch thickness)
- 1 cooking spray
- 1/4 cup of prepared basil pesto
- 1 thick slice of mozzarella cheese

DIRECTIONS

- Preheat the oven to 350 degrees.
- Spray a baking dish using cooking spray.
- Spread 2 tablespoons of the pesto sauce onto each flattened chicken breast.
- Place 1 slice of the cheese over the pesto.
- Roll up tightly and secure with toothpicks.
- Place in a lightly greased baking dish.
- Bake uncovered for about 45 minutes in the preheated oven, till juices run clear and chicken is nicely browned.
- Serve and enjoy.

CAESAR CHICKEN

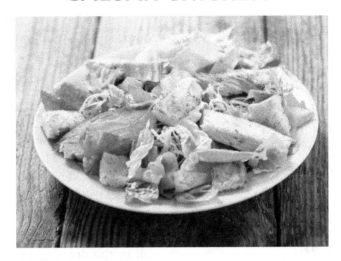

Caesar Salad is the kind of salad that can be eaten for lunch, dinner, side dish, and appetizer. It's sirtfood and keto-friendly as well. This recipe acts like a good protein source that our body needs for building muscles and tissues.

It provides some essential nutrients and fiber as well.

PREP TIME: 5 mins
COOK TIME: 10 min
TOTAL TIME: 15 mins
YIELD: 1 serving

NUTRITIONAL INFO

Calories: 674 cal | **Total fat:** 61 g | **Sugar:** 0 g | **Iron:** 0 mg | **Cholesterol:** 0 mg | **Carbohydrates:** 12 g | **Protein:** 20 g | **Fiber:** 5 g | **Calcium:** 0 mg | **Sodium:** 0 mg

INGREDIENTS

- 40 grams of Bacon Cubes
- 3 tablespoons of Olive oil (extra virgin)
- 1 tablespoon of Lemon juice
- 1 teaspoon of Mustard Yellow
- 1 1/2 pieces of Anchovy fillet
- 50 grams of Chicken breast
- 1 crop of Baby Romaine lettuce
- 1/2 piece of Cucumber

DIRECTIONS

- Cut the chicken fillet into strips.
- In a frying pan, fry the bacon cubes until crispy.
- Use a slotted spoon to remove them and leave the bacon fat in the pan.
- Fry the chicken strips all around the brown.
- Cook in the bacon fat inside the frying pan.
- Make the dressing in the meantime by mashing the olive oil, mustard, lemon juice, and anchovies into a smooth liquid.
- Chop the lettuce, mix in the cucumber, bacon, and chicken, then sprinkle with the dressing.
- Serve and enjoy.

PORK CARNITAS

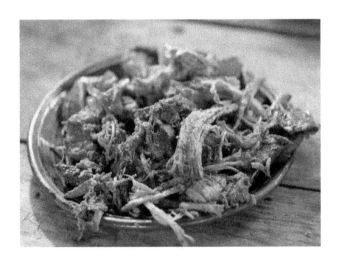

This recipe is perfect for lunch, dinner, and enjoyable as a side dish as well. Carnitas tends to be huge because it gives you a lot of meat that contains essential minerals such as iron, calcium, potassium, and sodium.

It as well provides high-quality protein, which will help your body to produce energy. Pork Carnitas offers a beautiful blend of flavors. So enjoy.

PREP TIME: 20 mins
COOK TIME: 8 hours
TOTAL TIME: 8 hours 20 mins
YIELD: 1 serving

NUTRITIONAL INFO

Calories: 254 cal | Total fat: 14 g | Sugar: 0 g | Iron: 0 mg | Cholesterol: 0 mg | Carbohydrates: 6 g | Protein: 26 g | Fiber: 1 g | Calcium: 0 mg | Sodium: 0 mg

INGREDIENTS

- 1/4 teaspoon of salt
- 1/4 piece of lime
- 125 grams of rib chop
- 1/2 piece of mango
- 1/4 piece of red onion
- 1/2 clove of garlic
- 1/4 tablespoon of paprika powder
- 1/4 teaspoon of cumin ground - grinded
- 1/4 teaspoon of chili powder

DIRECTIONS

- Cut the mango into cubes
- Chop the red onion
- Chop the garlic finely and squeeze the lime.
- Put the mango, garlic, and red onion in the slow cooker and place the rib chop on top.
- Rub the herbs into the meat
- Sprinkle with the lemon juice.
- Bring the slow cooker to a low setting.
- Cook the meat for about 8 hours.
- Use 2 forks to pull the meat apart.
- Heat a frying pan on medium-high heat.
- Fry the meat until it is a bit crispy.
- Serve with a crisp salad, guacamole, and/or tostones. They are so delicious.
- Enjoy.

MEATLOAF

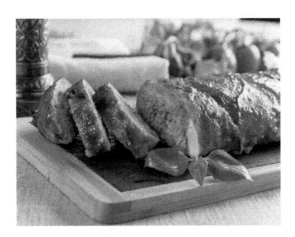

This is an easy recipe that won't take long to make at all. It's quite good for lunch. It features ground beef, egg, onion, dried bread crumbs, brown sugar, ketchup, and other healthy ingredients you need.

Meatloaf is full of protein and delightful flavors. It's mouthwatering and will never ruin your diet.

PREP TIME: 10 mins
COOK TIME: 1 hour
TOTAL TIME: 1 hour 10 mins
YIELD: 1 serving

NUTRITIONAL INFO

Calories: 372.1 cal | **Total fat:** 24.7 g | **Sugar:** 8.5 g | **Iron:** 2.4 mg | **Cholesterol:** 98 mg | **Carbohydrates:** 18.5 g | **Protein:** 18.2 g | **Fiber:** 1 g | **Calcium:** 80.5 mg | **Sodium:** 334.6 mg

INGREDIENTS

- 3/4 teaspoon of brown sugar
- 3/4 teaspoon of prepared mustard
- 2 teaspoons of ketchup
- 3 ounces of ground beef
- 1/8 egg
- 1/8 of chopped onion
- 2 tablespoons of dried bread crumbs
- salt and pepper to taste
- 2 tablespoons of milk

DIRECTIONS

- Preheat oven to 350 degrees F.
- Combine the egg, onion, egg, bread, and milk in a large bowl.
- Season with pepper and salt to taste.
- Place in a lightly greased 5 x 9-inch loaf pan.
- Combine the mustard, brown sugar, and ketchup in a separate small bowl.
- Mix well and pour over the meatloaf.
- Bake at 350 degrees F for an hour.
- Serve yourself and enjoy.

CARROT SALAD

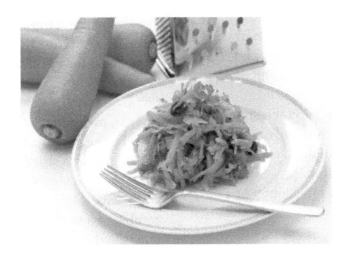

This is an undoubted carrot salad ever. It will become your to-go carrot salad recipe. Make sure you do not leave some ingredients out. It's tasty, crunchy, and highly nutritious.

Do you know they are a weight loss fast food that has been linked to improve your eye health and lower cholesterol levels in your body?

PREP TIME: 5 mins
COOK TIME: 0 min
TOTAL TIME: 5 mins
YIELD: 1 serving

NUTRITIONAL INFO

Calories: 229 cal | **Total fat:** 15 g | **Sugar:** 9 g | **Iron:** 1.3 mg | **Cholesterol:** 0 mg | **Carbohydrates:** 22 g | **Protein:** 3 g | **Fiber:** 4 g | **Calcium:** 31 mg | **Sodium:** 0 mg

INGREDIENTS

For the salad:
- 0.5 tablespoon of walnuts, chopped
- 0.5 tablespoon of pumpkin seeds
- 0.5-0.75 tablespoon of chopped parsley
- 1 medium carrot, grated
- 0.5 tablespoon of raisins
- 0.5 tablespoon of dried cranberries
- 0.5 tablespoon of unsweetened shredded coconut
- 0.5 tablespoon of pecans, chopped

For the dressing:
- 0.25 tablespoon of avocado oil
- 0.25 tablespoon of apple cider vinegar
- 0.25 teaspoon of unpasteurized honey
- 0.25 teaspoon of grated fresh ginger-root
- 0.13 teaspoon of Dijon mustard
- 0.06 teaspoon of salt
- 0.06 teaspoon of ground black pepper

DIRECTIONS

- In a large mixing bowl, combine all of the ingredients for the salad.
- Set it aside.
- Combine the apple cider vinegar, avocado oil, ginger-root, honey, salt, mustard and pepper in a small container and vigorously whisk with a fork until well combined and slightly emulsified.
- Pour over the reserved salad and toss well.
- Transfer into a serving bowl and garnish with grated coconut, more pumpkin seeds, and chopped parsley if you feel like.
- Serve immediately and enjoy.

CHICKEN CURRY

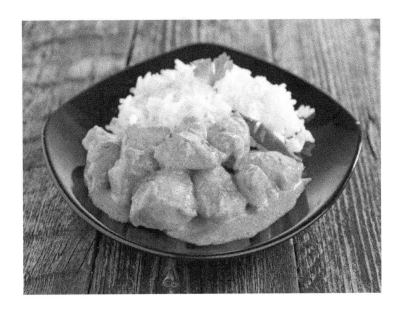

This is an adaptation of chicken curry from India. The flavors and aromas are a delight to the senses—smiles - so awesome.

It is best served with Basmati rice and Naan bread. It has some surprising health benefits: reducing inflammation, fighting cancer, and boosting your bones.

PREP TIME: 20 mins
COOK TIME: 25 mins
TOTAL TIME: 45 mins
YIELD: 1 serving

NUTRITIONAL INFO

Calories: 312.8 cal | **Total fat:** 21.7 g | **Sugar:** 6.7 g | **Iron:** 3.8 mg | **Cholesterol:** 37.9 mg | **Carbohydrates:** 14 g | **Protein:** 19.1 g | **Fiber:** 3.8 g | **Calcium:** 172.4 mg | **Sodium:** 268.3 mg

INGREDIENTS

- 3/4 teaspoon of tomato paste
- 1/4 cup of plain yogurt
- 3 tablespoons of coconut milk
- 1/8 juiced lemon
- 1/8 teaspoon of cayenne pepper
- 2-1/4 teaspoons of olive oil
- 1/4 chopped small onion
- 1/2 clove garlic, minced
- 1/8 teaspoon of grated fresh ginger root
- 1/8 teaspoon of white sugar
- 1/4 teaspoon of salt to taste
- 1/2 skinless, boneless chicken breast halves - cut into bite-size pieces
- 2-1/4 teaspoons of curry powder
- 1/4 teaspoon of ground cinnamon
- 1/4 teaspoon of paprika
- 1/4 bay leaf

DIRECTIONS

- In a skillet, heat olive oil over medium heat.
- Sauté onion until lightly browned.
- Stir in curry powder, garlic, paprika, cinnamon, ginger, bay leaf, salt, and sugar.
- Continue stirring for about 2 minutes.
- Add tomato paste, chicken pieces, coconut milk, yogurt.
- Bring to a boil and reduce heat.
- Simmer for about 20 minutes.
- Remove the bay leaf and stir in cayenne pepper and lemon juice.
- Simmer for another 5 minutes.
- Serve and enjoy.

CHICKEN FLAUTAS

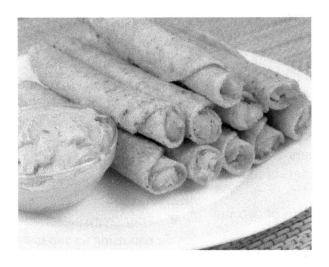

If you know how good it tastes, you'll be surprised.

The beautiful thing about this delicious food is that it's baked and easy to prepare.

PREP TIME: 10 mins
COOK TIME: 25 mins
TOTAL TIME: 35 mins
YIELD: 1 serving

NUTRITIONAL INFO

Calories: 448 cal | **Total fat:** 24 g | **Sugar:** 0 g | **Iron:** 0 mg | **Cholesterol:** 0 mg | **Carbohydrates:** 34 g | **Protein:** 24 g | **Fiber:** 8 g | **Calcium:** 0 mg | **Sodium:** 0 mg

INGREDIENTS

Tortillas:
- 1 piece of egg
- 2 tablespoons of almond milk
- 1/4 tablespoon of coconut oil
- 1 piece of satay skewers
- 20 grams of tapioca flour
- 10 grams of coconut flour
- 1/4 teaspoon of Celtic sea salt
- 1/4 teaspoon of garlic powder

Chicken Filling:
- 1/2 tablespoon of fresh coriander
- 1/2 tablespoon of jalapeno chili powder
- 50 grams of tomato cubes
- 1/4 piece of green pepper
- 1/2 cloves of garlic
- 1/4 piece of onion
- 1/4 tablespoon of coconut oil
- 65 ml of chicken stock
- 1/2 piece of chicken breast

DIRECTIONS

Making the tortillas:
- In a large bowl with a hand mixer, mix all of the ingredients except for the coconut oil until you have a smooth and zero batter.
- Put 1 tablespoon of coconut oil into the pan.
- Heat on a low medium high heat.
- Pour some batter into the pan using a soup ladle and fry a tortilla on both sides as if you're making an omelet.
- Take out the pan and put it on a plate.
- Repeat this till the batter is finished.

Making the filling:
- Snip the onion and cut the garlic cloves and jalapeno chili pepper finely.
- Dice the tomato, peel, and destone the avocado.
- Bring the chicken stock to the boil and then cook the chicken breast until done.
- Take the chicken out of the pan and allow it to cool before cutting it up into small cubes.

✗114

- salt and black pepper to taste

Guacamole:
- 1/4 piece of red onion
- 1/2 piece of lemon juice
- 1/4 piece of tomatoes
- 1/2 piece of avocado
- Salt and black pepper to taste

- In a frying pan, heat about 1/2 tablespoon of coconut oil and glaze the garlic and onion.
- Add the tomato, green pepper, and chili pepper.
- Fry for some minutes.
- Stir the chicken through the mixture.
- Use pepper and salt to season to taste.
- Get your tortilla ready.
- Place about 2 tablespoons of the filling on to the tortilla.
- Roll them up and use a pick to hold them together.
- Repeat for the rest of the tortillas.
- In a large frying pan, heat 1 tablespoon of coconut oil and fry the tortilla rolls.
- Serve with guacamole.
- Garnish with the fresh coriander.
- Enjoy.

TUNA STUFFED AVOCADO

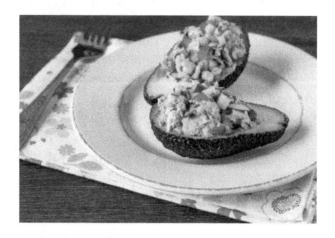

This recipe is so great for experimenting with a variety of different spices, vegetables, and vinegar.

It's quick and easy to prepare and packed with mayonnaise, balsamic vinegar, bell pepper, avocados, green onions, and some other healthy ingredients.

PREP TIME: 20 mins
COOK TIME: 25 mins
TOTAL TIME: 45 mins
YIELD: 1 serving

NUTRITIONAL INFO

Calories: 294 cal | **Total fat:** 18.2 g | **Sugar:** 2 g | **Iron:** 2 mg | **Cholesterol:** 27 mg | **Carbohydrates:** 11 g | **Protein:** 23.4 g | **Fiber:** 7.4 g | **Calcium:** 33 mg | **Sodium:** 154 mg

INGREDIENTS

- 1/4 dash of balsamic vinegar
- black pepper to taste
- 1/4 pinch of garlic salt, or to taste
- 1/2 ripe avocados, pitted and halved
- 1/4 (12 ounces) can of solid white tuna packed in water, drained
- 3/4 tablespoon of mayonnaise
- 3/4 green onions, thinly sliced, plus additional for garnish
- 1/8 chopped red bell pepper

DIRECTIONS

- In a bowl, stir together mayonnaise, tuna, red pepper, green onions, and balsamic vinegar.
- Season with garlic salt and pepper.
- Pack the tuna mixture with the avocado halves.
- Garnish with a dash of black pepper and the reserved green onions before serving.
- Serve and enjoy.

CHILLI CORN CARNE

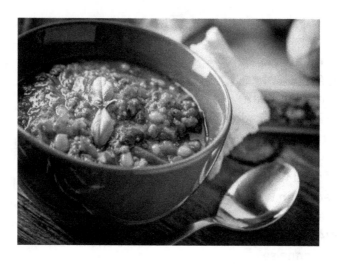

Adding a teaspoon of demerara sugar to this recipe will bring out the richness of the other spices. It is a portion of tasty comfort food that will help you reach the recommended daily dietary fiber goal.

This recipe helps in reducing the risk of heart disease, obesity, and type 2 diabetes. I hope you enjoy it.

PREP TIME: 20 mins
COOK TIME: 20 mins
TOTAL TIME: 40 mins
YIELD: 1 serving

NUTRITIONAL INFO

Calories: 301 cal | **Total fat:** 6 g | **Sugar:** 5.1 g | **Iron:** 4 mg | **Cholesterol:** 0 mg | **Carbohydrates:** 38.5 g | **Protein:** 11.5 g | **Fiber:** 10.6 g | **Calcium:** 66 mg | **Sodium:** 12 mg

INGREDIENTS

- 1/2 cube of beef stock
- 1 teaspoon of chili powder
- 1/4 teaspoon of drinking chocolate
- 1/2 teaspoon of mixed herbs
- 1 teaspoon of olive oil
- 1 small tin chopped tomatoes ; (200grams)
- 1 teaspoon of tomato puree
- 100 grams of lean minced beef
- 45 grams of kidney beans; drained canned
- 1/2 medium clove garlic
- 1/2 medium Onion
- 1/2 medium green pepper

DIRECTIONS

- In a non-stick saucepan, heat the olive oil and cook the onion until slightly softened.
- Add the diced pepper and garlic, then cook for some minutes.
- Add the minced beef, brown and drain off excess fat.
- Stir in the rest of the ingredients, adding chili powder to your taste.
- Cover and cook for about 20 minutes.
- Serve with brown rice.
- Enjoy.

ZOODLES WITH SHRIMP FLORENTINE

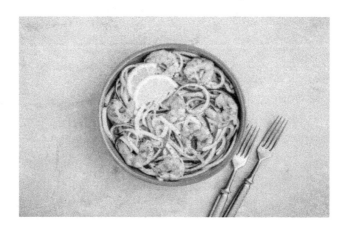

This is a quick, healthy, leisurely shrimp lunch made with zoodles instead of pasta. The ingredients here in this recipe are much, but they are healthy and can be found in the kitchen.

This recipe is the perfect choice if you're looking for a delicious low-carb meal.

PREP TIME: 10 mins
COOK TIME: 15 mins
TOTAL TIME: 25 mins
YIELD: 1 serving

NUTRITIONAL INFO

Calories: 229.2 cal | Total fat: 13.4 g | Sugar: 2.2 g | Iron: 4.3 mg | Cholesterol: 195.5 mg | Carbohydrates: 7.1 g | Protein: 21 g | Fiber: 12.3 g | Calcium: 99.9 mg | Sodium: 780.7 mg

INGREDIENTS

- 1/4 teaspoon of red pepper flakes
- 1/8 teaspoon of kosher salt
- 1/8 teaspoon of freshly ground black pepper
- 1/4 teaspoon of minced garlic
- 1/8 teaspoon of kosher salt
- 1-1/2 teaspoons of butter
- 1/4 pound of a large shrimp, peeled and deveined
- 1/4 teaspoon of minced garlic
- 1-1/2 teaspoons of butter
- 3/4 teaspoon of extra-virgin olive oil
- 1/2 zucchini, cut into noodle-shape strands
- 1/8 large yellow onion, minced
- 3/4 teaspoon of fresh lemon juice
- 1/4 (6 ounces) bag of baby spinach

DIRECTIONS

- In a large skillet over medium heat, heat olive oil and 1 tablespoon of butter.
- Cook and stir in zoodles, chopped garlic, onion, and 1/1 teaspoon of salt for about 5 minutes, until zoodles are tender and onion is translucent.
- Transfer zoodles mixture into a bowl.
- In the same skillet, heat about 2 tablespoons of butter.
- Cook and stir minced garlic and shrimp for about 3 to 4 minutes, until shrimp are just pink.
- Add lemon juice, spinach, red pepper flakes, pepper, and 1/2 teaspoon of salt.
- Cook and stir for about 3 minutes, until spinach starts to wilt.
- Add zoodle mixture and cook and stir for about 2 minutes, until heated through.
- Serve and enjoy.

TOMATO SALSA

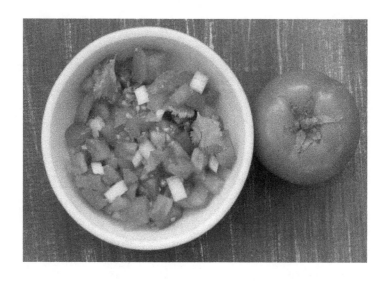

This is a delicious homemade salsa. This recipe is a good dose of vitamin c, and it can stabilize your blood sugar.

They are a fantastic salsa, and they taste great with a clove of chopped
garlic.

PREP TIME: 10 mins
ADDITIONAL TIME: 1 hour
TOTAL TIME: 1 hour 10 mins
YIELD: 1 serving

NUTRITIONAL INFO

Calories: 51.5 cal | **Total fat:** 0.2 g | **Sugar:** 3.4 g | **Iron:** 0.4 mg | **Cholesterol:** 0 mg | **Carbohydrates:** 3.7 g | **Protein:** 2.1 g | **Fiber:** 3.7 g | **Calcium:** 18.4 mg |

INGREDIENTS

- 3/4 of chopped tomatoes
- 2 tablespoons of chopped fresh cilantro
- 1/4 teaspoon of salt
- 1/2 teaspoon of lime juice
- 2 tablespoons of finely diced onion
- 1-1/4 serrano chiles, finely chopped

DIRECTIONS

- Stir together onion, chili peppers, tomatoes, salt, cilantro, and lime juice in a medium bowl.
- Chill for about an hour in the refrigerator before serving.
- Serve and enjoy.

SHAKSHUKA

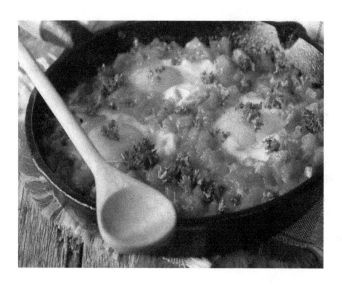

You will love this recipe because it's healthy, easy, and satisfying. You can make this with jalapeno and fresh tomato whenever you want to prepare your meal.

Enjoy.

PREP TIME: 10 mins
COOK TIME: 35 mins
TOTAL TIME: 45 mins
YIELD: 1 serving

NUTRITIONAL INFO

Calories: 293.5 cal | **Total fat:** 9.4 g | **Sugar:** 7.7 g | **Iron:** 4.5 mg | **Cholesterol:** 186 mg | **Carbohydrates:** 40.9 g | **Protein:** 13.1 g | **Fiber:** 4.3 g | **Calcium:** 143.8 mg | **Sodium:** 654.2 mg

INGREDIENTS

- 3/4 teaspoon of olive oil
- 1/4 teaspoon of paprika, or to taste
- 1/2 slice pickled jalapeno pepper, finely chopped
- 1 egg
- 1/2 clove of minced garlic
- 1/4 onion, cut into 2 inch pieces
- 1/4 (28 ounces) can whole of peeled plum tomatoes with juice
- 1/4 green bell pepper, cut into 2-inch pieces
- 1 (6 inches) pita bread - optional

DIRECTIONS

- In a deep skillet, heat the vegetable oil over medium heat.
- Stir in onion, garlic, and bell pepper.
- Cook and stir for about 5 minutes, until the onion has turned translucent and softened.
- Add the paprika, canned tomatoes, jalapenos, and paprika.
- Stir and break up the tomatoes using the back of a spoon.
- Simmer for 25 minutes.
- In a small bowl, crack an egg and then slip the egg into the tomato sauce gently.
- Repeat this with the rest of the eggs.
- Cook the eggs for about 2 to 3 minutes, until the yolks have thickened but not hard and whites are firm.
- Add a little tablespoon of water if the tomato sauce gets dry.
- Use a slotted spoon to remove the eggs and place onto a warm plate.
- Serve with the pita bread and tomato sauce.
- Enjoy.

BRAISED CABBAGE

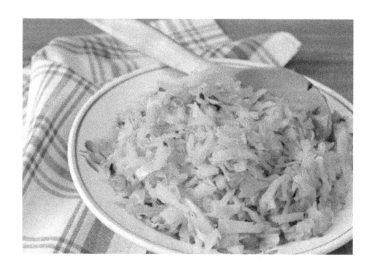

Having this meal would turn out to be delightful. It's a basic substantial cabbage dish that is better than boiled and not as greasy as fried.

The caraway seeds and vinegar sugar add good flavor and a bit of tanginess to it. You can add garlic as well or maybe, throw in sliced carrots for color.

You would love it because it's spectacularly good for you.

PREP TIME: 10 mins
COOK TIME: 25 mins
TOTAL TIME: 35 mins
YIELD: 1 serving

NUTRITIONAL INFO

Calories: 76.5 cal | **Total fat:** 4.1 g | **Sugar:** 6 g | **Iron:** 0.6 mg | **Cholesterol:** 10.2 mg | **Carbohydrates:** 9.9 g | **Protein:** 1.6 g | **Fiber:** 3 g | **Calcium:** 51.1 mg | **Sodium:** 434.6 mg

INGREDIENTS

- 1/2 teaspoon of white sugar
- 1/4 teaspoon of caraway seeds
- 1/8 teaspoon of salt
- 1 teaspoon of butter, or more to taste
- 1/8 head cabbage, cored and cut into 1/4-inch slices
- 1/8 onion, cut into 1/4-inch slices
- 2 tablespoons and 2 teaspoons of water
- 1/2 teaspoon of white vinegar

DIRECTIONS

- In a large skillet over medium heat, melt butter.
- Cook and stir cabbage and onion for about 5 minutes, until onions are translucent.
- Pour in water, add sugar, vinegar, salt, and caraway seeds.
- Reduce heat to low and cook, stirring occasionally, for about 20 minutes, until cabbage is tender.
- Serve and enjoy.

INDIAN SHRIMP CURRY

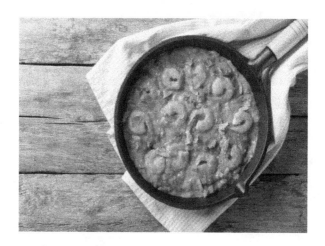

You're lucky to have found this recipe in this book.

This recipe has an authentic taste and a straightforward meal to prepare whenever you're in haste. You'll be using a skillet for this recipe.

So before adding the shrimp to skillet, make sure you pop the shrimp tails off and serve with rice.

PREP TIME: 15 mins
COOK TIME: 15 mins
TOTAL TIME: 30 mins
YIELD: 1 serving

NUTRITIONAL INFO

Calories: 416.2 cal | Total fat: 32.1 g | Sugar: 3.5 g | Iron: 8.8 mg | Cholesterol: 146 mg | Carbohydrates: 10.9 g | Protein: 23 g | Fiber: 2.9 g | Calcium: 119.2 mg | Sodium: 930.4 mg

INGREDIENTS

- 1/4 teaspoon of ground cumin
- 1/8 teaspoon of ground turmeric
- 1/4 teaspoon of paprika
- 1/4 pound of cooked and peeled shrimp
- 1-1/2 teaspoons of chopped fresh cilantro
- 1/8 teaspoon of red chili powder
- 1/4 (14.5 ounce) can of chopped tomatoes
- 1/4 (14 ounce) can of coconut milk
- 1-1/2 teaspoons of peanut oil
- 1/8 minced sweet onion
- 1/2 clove garlic, chopped
- 1/4 teaspoon of ground ginger
- 1/4 teaspoon of salt

DIRECTIONS

- In a large skillet, heat the oil over medium heat.
- Cook the onion in the hot oil for about 5 minutes, until translucent.
- Remove the skillet from the heat and allow it to cool for 2 mins.
- Add the ginger, garlic, cumin, paprika, turmeric, and ground chili to the onion and stir over low heat.
- Pour the coconut milk and tomatoes into the skillet.
- Season with salt.
- Cook the mixture at a simmer, stirring occasionally, for 10 mins.
- Stir the fresh cilantro, shrimp, and dried cilantro into the sauce mixture.
- Cook for another 1 minute before serving.
- Serve and enjoy.

SWEET POTATO HASH

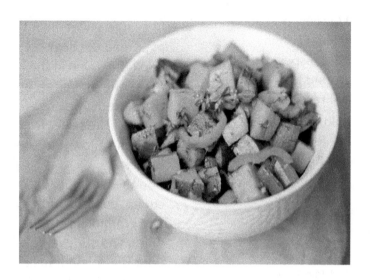

Sweet Potato Hash is a delicious, versatile, healthy, and vegetarian full meal you can have for lunch. It's so amazing and yummy, and it lasts forever in the pantry.

They are even healthier than all these white potatoes out there. These Potatoes can go savory or sweet. So amazing.

What I love about this recipe is that they are packed with nutrition.

PREP TIME: 10 mins
COOK TIME: 25 mins
TOTAL TIME: 35 mins
YIELD: 1 serving

NUTRITIONAL INFO

Calories: 157 cal | **Total fat:** 7 g | **Sugar:** 5 g | **Iron:** 0.6 mg | **Cholesterol:** 146 mg | **Carbohydrates:** 0 g | **Protein:** 1 g | **Fiber:** 3 g | **Calcium:** 43 mg | **Sodium:** 942 mg

INGREDIENTS

- 0.5 stalks celery, diced
- 0.38 teaspoon of sea salt
- 0.13 teaspoon of ground black pepper
- 0.5 tablespoon of olive oil
- 0.75 medium sweet potatoes, skin-on and diced into equal, bite-size chunks
- 0.13 medium white onion, diced
- 0.5 cloves garlic, minced
- sliced green onions, for garnish

DIRECTIONS

- In a large pan over medium-high heat, heat oil.
- Add the onion, potatoes, and celery to the oil and then sprinkle with pepper and salt.
- Stir to combine, cover and cook until the potatoes are almost tender, for about 15 minutes, stirring occasionally.
- Turn the heat to high.
- Add the garlic and stir to combine.
- Cook on high until sweet potatoes are nicely browned, for about 2 to 5 minutes.
- Serve hot with sliced green onions if you feel like.
- Enjoy.

CAULIFLOWER FRITTERS

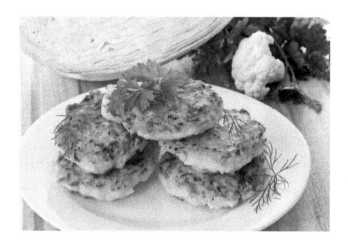

Cauliflower Fritters are a different way to have cauliflower and easy to make. They are so tasty and delicious as well.

A recipe you'll make several times without getting tired of it. They are flexible and just so good for you. You can make as your main dish with a side salad.

PREP TIME: 10 mins
COOK TIME: 10 mins
TOTAL TIME: 20 mins
YIELD: 1 serving

NUTRITIONAL INFO

Calories: 129.7 cal | **Total fat:** 4.9 g | **Sugar:** 4.3 g | **Iron:** 1.5 mg | **Cholesterol:** 107.9 mg | **Carbohydrates:** 15.3 g | **Protein:** 6.7 g | **Fiber:** 2.8 g | **Calcium:** 84 mg | **Sodium:** 682.2 mg

INGREDIENTS

- 1/2 extra-large eggs
- 1/8 teaspoon of baking powder
- 1 cup of cauliflower florets
- 1 tablespoon and 1 teaspoon of all-purpose flour
- 1/8 (7 ounce) package of dry Italian-style salad dressing mix
- 1 tablespoon and 1 teaspoon of olive oil for frying, or as needed

DIRECTIONS

- In a food processor finely minced, process cauliflower.
- Transfer into a large bowl.
- Stir eggs, flour, Italian dressing mix, and baking powder into the cauliflower.
- Heat enough olive oil over medium heat to cover the bottom of a frying pan.
- Drop heaping tablespoons of the cauliflower mixture into the hot oil.
- Fry for about 3 minutes per side until golden brown.
- Serve and enjoy.

DATE AND BACON APPETIZER

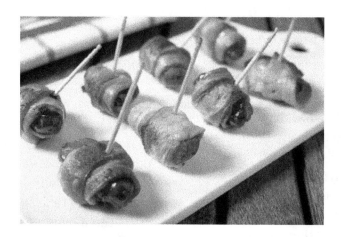

These Dates are stuffed with almonds and can be wrapped in bacon. They are a quick and easy appetizer you can have when sunset. You'll feel the joy in you. It would be so beautiful.

They would come out great when baked at 400 for a little longer than broiling them. I bet you; they cook a little more evenly. By the way, they are a hit when served at parties.

PREP TIME: 30 mins
COOK TIME: 5 mins
TOTAL TIME: 35 mins
YIELD: 1 serving

NUTRITIONAL INFO

Calories: 559.7 cal | **Total fat:** 43.7 g | **Sugar:** 24.5 g | **Iron:** 1.5 mg | **Cholesterol:** 51.5 mg | **Carbohydrates:** 32.2 g | **Protein:** 13.7 g | **Fiber:** 5.2 g | **Calcium:** 65.4 mg | **Sodium:** 631.1 mg

INGREDIENTS

- 2-1/2 ounces of sliced bacon
- 1/8 (8 ounce) package of pitted dates
- 1/2 ounce of almonds

DIRECTIONS

- Preheat the broiler
- Slit dates and place 1 almond inside each date.
- Wrap the dates with bacon and use toothpicks to hold them together.
- Broil until bacon is evenly crisp and brown, for about 10 minutes.
- Serve and enjoy.

ENSALADA RUSA

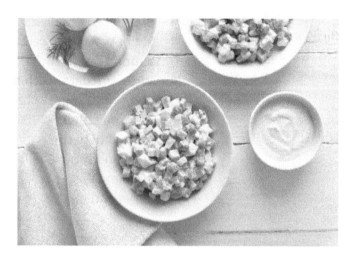

The beets and the color will conjure great interest during your lunch.

You'll love it the first time you try it. They are so delicious.

Give this recipe a try if you're looking for a variation on ordinary potato salad. You won't regret it at all.

PREP TIME: 20 mins
COOK TIME: 20 mins
ADDITIONAL TIME: 20 mins
TOTAL TIME: 1 hr 40 mins
YIELD: 1 serving

NUTRITIONAL INFO

Calories: 459.4 cal | Total fat: 27.1 g | Sugar: 6.5 g | Iron: 3.1 mg | Cholesterol: 196.4 mg | Carbohydrates: 44.3 g | Protein: 11.8 g | Fiber: 6.4 g | Calcium: 64.2 mg | Sodium: 868.3 mg

INGREDIENTS

- 1/4 teaspoon of salt
- 1 egg
- 3/4 trimmed beets
- 1 potato, peeled and cubed
- 2 tablespoons of mayonnaise, or to taste

DIRECTIONS

- In a saucepan, place the beets and cover with water, then bring to a boil.
- Reduce the heat to medium and boil gently for about 20 minutes, until tender.
- Remove from the boiling water and let it cool.
- Peel and dice the beets. Then chill.
- In a separate saucepan, place the potatoes and add water to cover.
- Stir in salt and boil the potato cubes for about 15 minutes, until tender but not mushy.
- Drain the potatoes in colander set in the sink. Chill as well.
- Bring a saucepan of water to a boil and reduce heat to medium.
- Stir in 1 or 2 teaspoons of salt.
- Gently lower the eggs into the boiling water. Make sure they don't hit the bottom of the pan.
- Crack and simmer for about 15 minutes.
- Remove the eggs to a bowl filled with ice water and ice.
- Let the eggs chill till cold thoroughly.
- Peel and dice the eggs.
- In a salad bowl, mix the potato cubes, chilled beets, and eggs together.
- Gently stir in mayonnaise to taste.
- Serve and enjoy.

SHRIMP WITH SCRAMBLED EGGS

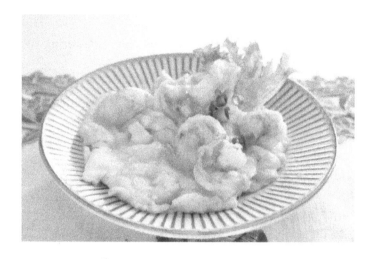

Shrimp with Scrambled eggs is a typical dish that you always sure to order. There's something about these silky scrambled eggs and tender shrimp that makes it a must-order.

So you need to prepare it yourself today for lunch and don't spend extra money to place order for this dish. They are so beautiful and delicious. Just follow the recipe given and enjoy it.

PREP TIME: 5 mins
COOK TIME: 5 mins
TOTAL TIME: 10 mins
YIELD: 1 serving

NUTRITIONAL INFO

Calories: 245 cal | **Total fat:** 12 g | **Sugar:** 0 g | **Iron:** 0 mg | **Cholesterol:** 566 mg | **Carbohydrates:** 3 g | **Protein:** 29 g | **Fiber:** 0 g | **Calcium:** 121 mg | **Sodium:** 1050 mg

INGREDIENTS

- 1/4 cup of chicken broth or stock
- Up to 1/8 teaspoon of salt
- 2 tablespoons of oil for frying
- Pepper to taste
- 1/2 teaspoon of Chinese rice wine or dry sherry
- 1 teaspoon of oyster sauce
- 1 green onion, thinly sliced on the diagonal
- 4 ounces of shrimp, deveined and peeled (**Note:** Cut the shrimp if they are too large.)
- 4 large eggs, lightly beaten

DIRECTIONS

- Bring together all of the ingredients.
- Wash the shrimp and pat dry it.
- Take beaten eggs and stir in the salt, chicken broth, pepper, oyster sauce, rice wine, and green onion.
- Add 1 tablespoon of oil to a preheated skillet or wok.
- Add the shrimp when the oil is hot.
- Stir-fry until they turn pink.
- Remove and drain.
- Add 1 tablespoon of oil.
- Turn the heat on high and add the egg mixture when the oil is hot.
- Gently scramble for 1 minute, then add the shrimp.
- Continue scrambling till the eggs are almost cooked till moist.
- Remove the heat. Let it sit for 1 minute.
- Serve and enjoy.

Dinner
Recipes

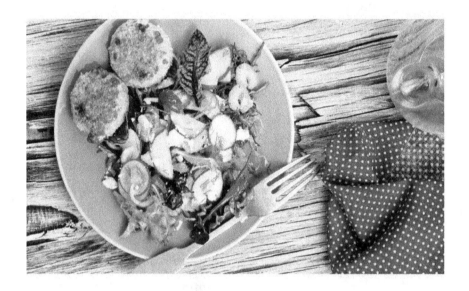

Adele Bayles

140

VEGGIE STIR-FRY WITH SOBA NOODLE

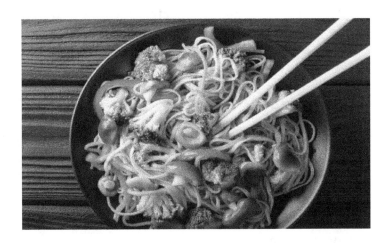

This is an easy and quick meal for a single person, and perfect as a sirtfood, dairy-free, and vegetarian dinner.

This recipe is for you if you love ordering noodles from Chinese takeout.

This Veggie Stir Fry With Soba Noodle is hugely better than takeout because it's loaded with veggies and lighter than most Chinese takeout dishes. I hope you love it when you're ready to prepare it.

PREP TIME: 5 mins
COOK TIME: 10 mins
TOTAL TIME: 15 mins
YIELD: 1 serving

NUTRITIONAL INFO

Calories: 488 cal | Total fat: 21 g | Sugar: 4 g | Iron: 0 mg | Cholesterol: 186 mg | Carbohydrates: 63.5 g | Protein: 18.5 g | Fiber: 4 g | Calcium: 0 mg | Sodium: 1120 mg

INGREDIENTS

- 1/4 cup of broccoli florets
- 1 large pasture-raised egg
- 1 tablespoon of coconut aminos
- 1 tablespoon of Sriracha sauce, or less if you don't like it too spicy
- 1 tablespoon of creamy nut butter
- 2 ounces of uncooked soba noodles
- 1/2 tablespoon of toasted sesame oil
- 1/2 teaspoon of minced garlic
- 1/2 teaspoon of ground ginger
- 1/4 cup of chopped onion
- 1/4 cup of chopped bell pepper

DIRECTIONS

- Add water into medium water and bring it to a boil.
- Add the soba noodles and cook for about 4 to 6 minutes, until tender.
- Heat the sesame oil in a large skillet over medium heat. Do this while the noodles cook.
- Add the onion, garlic, ginger, broccoli, and bell pepper.
- Cover the skillet and cook, stirring occasionally, for about 3 to 4 minutes, until softened.
- Strain the soba noodles and add them to the vegetables in the skillet.
- Push everything to a side and crack the egg into the skillet.
- Cook, breaking up the white and yolk until scrambled, then mix into the noodles and vegetables.
- Add the sriracha, coconut aminos, and nut butter and mix well.
- Serve warm and enjoy.

ASPARAGUS WITH PRAWN TAGLIATELLE

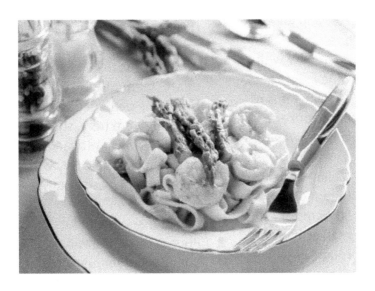

This is a quick Asparagus With Prawn Tagliatelle dish that is ready within 15 minutes. You can quickly bulk it up with some cream fraiche and some new nests of pasta.

PREP TIME: 5 mins
COOK TIME: 10 mins
TOTAL TIME: 15 mins
YIELD: 1 serving

NUTRITIONAL INFO

Calories: 574 cal | **Total fat:** 11 g | **Sugar:** 5 g | **Iron:** 0 mg | **Cholesterol:** 0 mg | **Carbohydrates:** 75 g | **Protein:** 30 g | **Fiber:** 10 g | **Calcium:** 0 mg | **Sodium:** 0 mg

INGREDIENTS

- 2-3 garlic cloves, crushed
- zest and juice of 1 lemon
- 100ml dry white wine
- 1 x 150grams of pack cooked king prawns
- 3 nests of dried tagliatelle (about 195g)
- 50grams of regular broccoli, roughly chopped
- 10grams of butter
- 125grams of asparagus, trimmed and roughly chopped
- 3/4 x 15grams pack of flat-leaf parsley, leaves chopped.

DIRECTIONS

- In a large pan, bring salted water to the boil.
- Drop in the pasta nests and cook for about 6 minutes
- Add the broccoli and cook until al dente, for another 3 minutes.
- In a frying pan, melt the butter over medium heat, stirring until it starts to smell nutty and until it's speckled with color brown.
- Add the garlic, asparagus, and half the lemon juice.
- Cook for some minutes.
- Pour in the white wine.
- Stir all together and simmer until the asparagus is almost tender and the wine has bubbled away by half, for about 2 minutes.
- Stir in the prawns and heat through.
- Drain the broccoli and tagliatelle. Save a splash of pasta water.
- Toss with the asparagus and garlicky prawns, adding little of pasta water to create a coating.
- Stir through the parsley, extra lemon juice, and the lemon zest, to taste.
- Season with black pepper, then serve in warmed bowls.
- Scattered with the remaining lemon zest.
- Enjoy.

✗144

GRILLED VEGETABLES

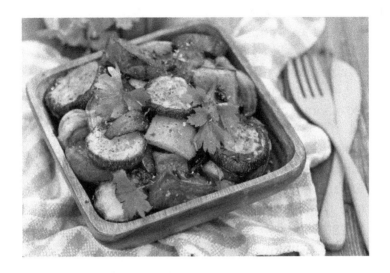

Vegetables with the simple additions of freshly ground black pepper, kosher salt, and extra virgin olive oil taste incredible when grilled.

They will probably need more salt than you think and you can cook them in a frying pan instead of grilling, and maybe use any combination of the following veggies if you want.

PREP TIME: 20 mins
COOK TIME: 10 mins
TOTAL TIME: 30 mins
YIELD: 1 serving

NUTRITIONAL INFO

Calories: 210.4 cal | **Total fat:** 19.1 g | **Sugar:** 3.5 g | **Iron:** 0.8 mg | **Cholesterol:** 0 mg | **Carbohydrates:** 8.8 g | **Protein:** 2.8 g | **Fiber:** 2.5 g | **Calcium:** 21.7 mg | **Sodium:** 80.5 mg

INGREDIENTS

- 1/8 red onion, cut into 1/2-inch-thick slices
- 1 tablespoon and 1-1/4 teaspoons of extra-virgin olive oil
- 1 pinch of kosher salt to taste
- 3/8 zucchinis, cut into 1/2-inch slices
- 3/8 green bell peppers, cut into chunks
- 1-1/2 ounces of whole button mushrooms
- 1-1/2 ounces of cherry tomatoes
- 1 pinch of freshly ground black pepper to taste

DIRECTIONS

- Preheat an outdoor grill for medium-high heat.
- Lightly oil the grate.
- Combine together green bell peppers, zucchinis, tomatoes, mushrooms, and onion in a large bowl.
- Pour olive oil over the vegetables and then toss to evenly coat.
- Season with pepper and salt.
- Grill vegetables on preheated grill for about 3 to 5 minutes per side, until lightly charred.
- Serve and enjoy.

SPICY POTATO CURRY

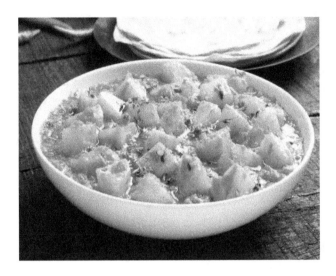

This spicy potato curry is packed with abundant spices, which makes it better than any restaurant curry. It completely spots on, giving a very authentic and rich flavor with the right amount of spiciness.

The curry is also good with spinach in it.

PREP TIME: 30 mins
COOK TIME: 30 mins
TOTAL TIME: 1 hour
YIELD: 1 serving

NUTRITIONAL INFO

Calories: 406.9 cal | **Total fat:** 20.1 g | **Sugar:** 5.9 g | **Iron:** 7 mg | **Cholesterol:** 0 mg | **Carbohydrates:** 50.6 g | **Protein:** 10.1 g | **Fiber:** 10.1 g | **Calcium:** 106.7 mg | **Sodium:** 1175 mg

INGREDIENTS

- 1/4 teaspoon of ground cumin
- 1/4 teaspoon of cayenne pepper
- 3/4 teaspoon of curry powder
- 3/4 teaspoon of garam masala
- 1/8 (1 inch) piece fresh ginger root, peeled and minced
- 1/4 teaspoon salt
- 1/8 (15 ounce) can of peas, drained
- 1/8 (14 ounce) can of coconut milk
- 1/8 (14.5 ounce) can of diced tomatoes
- 5/8 potatoes, peeled and cubed
- 1 teaspoon of vegetable oil
- 1/8 yellow onion, diced
- 1/2 clove garlic, minced
- 1/8 (15 ounce) can of garbanzo beans (chickpeas), rinsed and drained

DIRECTIONS

- In a large pot, place potatoes with salted water.
- Bring to a boil over high heat.
- Reduce heat to medium-low, cover, and simmer for about 15 minutes, until just tender.
- Drain and allow to steam dry for a minute.
- In a large skillet, heat the vegetables over medium heat.
- Stir in the garlic and onion.
- Cook and stir for about 5 minutes, until the onion has softened and turned translucent.
- Season with cayenne pepper, cumin, curry powder, ginger, garam masala, and salt.
- Cook for another 2 minutes.
- Add the garbanzo beans, potatoes, tomatoes, and peas.
- Pour in the coconut milk and bring to a simmer.
- Simmer for about 5 - 10 minutes.
- Serve and enjoy.

STUFFED EGGPLANT

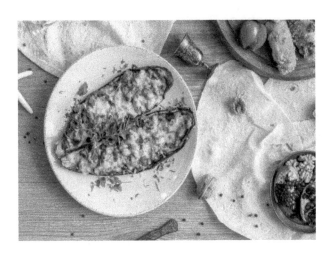

Stuffed Eggplant is delicious, and it is excellent as the main course, but you can buy the mini Eggplant and then use them as appetizer or side dish. This is a must-try!

It's advisable you reduce the breadcrumbs and don't chop Eggplant too much. I hope you enjoy it later when you prepare it. Enjoy.

PREP TIME: 30 mins
COOK TIME: 30 mins
TOTAL TIME: 1 hour
YIELD: 1 serving

NUTRITIONAL INFO

Calories: 976.5 cal | **Total fat:** 69.7 g | **Sugar:** 7.1 g | **Iron:** 5.1 mg | **Cholesterol:** 97.9 mg | **Carbohydrates:** 51.6 g | **Protein:** 31 g | **Fiber:** 7.7 g | **Calcium:** 289 mg | **Sodium:** 2082 mg

INGREDIENTS

- 1-1/2 teaspoons of chopped fresh parsley
- 2 tablespoons of white wine
- 1/2 cup of Italian seasoned bread crumbs
- 1/4 eggplant, halved lengthwise
- salt and pepper to taste
- 2 tablespoons of olive oil, divided
- 1/4 pound of sweet Italian sausage, casings removed
- 1/2 clove chopped garlic
- 2 tablespoons of grated Parmesan cheese, divided

DIRECTIONS

- Preheat oven to 350 degrees F
- Scoop out the flesh of the eggplant. Chop it and reserve.
- Season shells with pepper and salt, coat with some olive oil, and set it aside.
- In a large deep skillet, heat 1/4 cup of olive oil over medium-high heat.
- Sauté garlic and sausage until sausage is evenly brown.
- Stir in the reserved chopped eggplant.
- Season with pepper, parsley, and salt.
- Pour the wine in and cook for about 5 minutes.
- Mix in 1/4 cup of Parmesan cheese and bread crumbs.
- Stir in more olive oil if the mixture is dry.
- Stuff mixture into the eggplant shells.
- Sprinkle top with the rest of the Parmesan cheese.
- Bake in the preheated oven until eggplant is tender, for about 30 minutes.
- Serve and enjoy.

BROCCOLI WITH CHICKEN

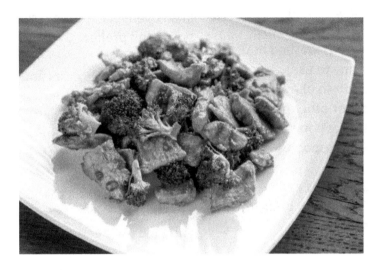

Broccoli with chicken is an excellent recipe that can be ready within 20 minutes. You have just 5 minutes of prep to make this dish for dinner.

There is zero better busy weeknight dinner than one that gives time to have a glass of wine while the dinner makes itself!

PREP TIME: 5 mins
COOK TIME: 15 mins
TOTAL TIME: 20 mins
YIELD: 1 serving

NUTRITIONAL INFO

Calories: 391 cal | **Total fat:** 13 g | **Sugar:** 1 g | **Iron:** 0 mg | **Cholesterol:** 165 mg | **Carbohydrates:** 5 g | **Protein:** 60 g | **Fiber:** 1 g | **Calcium:** 70 mg | **Sodium:** 636 mg

INGREDIENTS

- 1 pack Mann's Broccolini (they're already washed and ready to use)
- 1 splash of avocado oil (or other high smoke point oil)
- 2 tablespoons of butter
- 2-3 cloves garlic
- 2-3 chicken breasts
- sea salt
- Pepper
- fresh parsley (optional, for garnish)

DIRECTIONS

- In an oven, place your cast iron skillet and preheat to 450 degrees F.
- Pat dry chicken breasts and sprinkle salt and pepper generously on both sides.
- Crush garlic and add into a small pot with melt butter and butter.
- Add chicken breasts to the smoking hot skillet, broccolli, and then pour garlic butter over it.
- Bake for about 15 minutes.
- Remove from the oven and then let it rest for 5 minutes.
- Serve and sprinkle with freshly chopped parsley.
- Enjoy.

TOASTED PINE NUTS WITH GREEN KALE

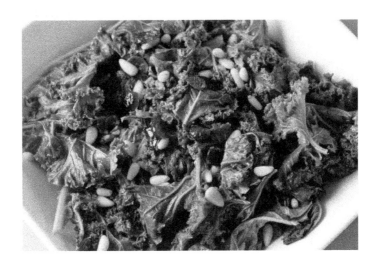

Toasted pine nuts with green kale are the best kale recipe you would ever try. You can use regular raisins and roasted almonds.

It's effortless to prepare, and you'll enjoy the sweetness of the raisins with kale.

PREP TIME: 5 mins
COOK TIME: 15 mins
TOTAL TIME: 20 mins
YIELD: 1 serving

NUTRITIONAL INFO

Calories: 319.8 cal | **Total fat:** 17.4 g | **Sugar:** 15 g | **Iron:** 0 mg | **Cholesterol:** 0 mg | **Carbohydrates:** 40.4 g | **Protein:** 9.1 g | **Fiber:** 0 g | **Calcium:** 0 mg | **Sodium:** 84.6 mg

INGREDIENTS

- 2 cups of water
- 4 garlic cloves, minced
- 1/3 cup of raisins
- 1/4 cup of toasted pine nuts
- 3/4 pound of green kale, washed, stems removed, and shredded
- 2 teaspoons of olive oil
- salt and pepper

DIRECTIONS

- Place the pine nuts on the cookie sheet for about 5 minutes in a 325 degrees F oven. You need to be careful. This is because they burn easily.
- In a skillet, bring water to a boil with a tight-fitting lid.
- Add kale and cook for about 5 minutes or until kale is just tender.
- Drain and set it aside.
- Rinse out the skillet.
- Dry and add olive oil.
- Heat over medium heat and add your garlic.
- Sauté for about 30 seconds.
- Add raisins and then stir for about 30 seconds.
- This time, the raisins should be slightly puffed and glossy.
- Add kale, stir and season.
- Sauté until heated through.
- Garnish with the pine nuts and then serve.
- Enjoy.

MUSHROOM WITH BOK CHOY

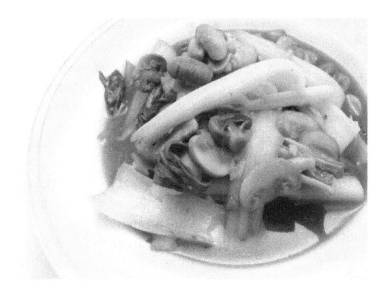

Mushroom with Bok Choy requires just 10 minutes to make and is best served with the main dinner dishes.

You can be creative with this dish by using any mushrooms for cooking bok choy: king trumpet, buna shimeji, white, cremini, enoki, oyster mushrooms, etc. You can as well combine some types of mushrooms to stir fry. It's totally up to you. The fact is the result will always be delectable.

PREP TIME: 8 mins
COOK TIME: 2 mins
TOTAL TIME: 10 mins
YIELD: 1 serving

NUTRITIONAL INFO

Calories: 135 cal | Total fat: 11 g | Sugar: 3 g | Iron: 1.4 mg | Cholesterol: 0 mg | Carbohydrates: 8 g | Protein: 4 g | Fiber: 0 g | Calcium: 157 mg | Sodium: 389 mg

INGREDIENTS

- 0.75 tablespoons of oil
- 2 ounces of shiitake mushrooms (stem removed and sliced)
- 5 ounces of bok choy (rinsed and drained)
- 1.5 cloves garlic, minced
- 0.13 teaspoon salt or to taste

DIRECTIONS

- Use cold water to rinse the bok choy, drained.
- Cut and remove the lower part of the bok choy stems.
- Cut the leaves lengthwise to halves and set it aside.
- Place a pan or wok on high heat.
- Add the oil until heated, add the garlic and then stir-fry until aromatic.
- Add the mushroom and do some quick stir before adding the bok choy.
- Add salt, then continue to stir fry till steams remain crisp, and leaves are wilted.
- Turn off the heat.
- Serve immediately and enjoy.

LAMB CHOPS WITH CRISPY KALE

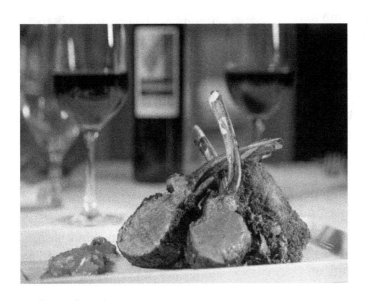

This is an elegant dinner that is made with lamb loin chops, capers, anchovy, and some other healthy and nutritious ingredients.

Serve your pile chops with crispy kale and enjoy everything with grilled lemon juice. You would love it!

PREP TIME: 10 mins
COOK TIME: 0 mins
TOTAL TIME: 10 mins
YIELD: 1 serving

NUTRITIONAL INFO

Calories: 900 cal | **Total fat:** 75.4 g | **Sugar:** 0.1 g | **Iron:** 24 mg | **Carbohydrates:** 4.1 g | **Protein:** 287.2 g | **Fiber:** 0.3 g

INGREDIENTS

- 12 lamb loin chops (buy medium-sized Frenched chops)
- 2 lemons
- 12 to 15 leaves sage, picked
- 1/2 cup of Virgin Olive Oil
- Salt and pepper
- 3 tablespoons of capers in brine, drained
- 6 fillets of anchovy in oil, drained
- 4 cloves garlic, crushed
- 1 large bunch Tuscan (flat) kale, cleaned, patted dry and

DIRECTIONS

- Pound each chop into 1/8 to 1/4 inch thick medallions attached to the bone.
- Season both sides of pounded chop with pepper and salt.
- Pile up the anchovies, capers, zest of 1 lemon, and garlic, then finely chop everything together. Mash it in a bit using the side of your knife.
- Pile the sage leaves on top of one another and then thinly slice.
- In a large plastic baggie, add paste and sage. Add olive oil and then mush to combine, then drop in chops and refrigerate for an hour over the night.
- Preheat oven to 500 degrees F.
- Set a wire rack into a rimmed baking sheet.
- Bring out the chops and let them come to room temperature.
- Spray the kale on both sides lightly and arrange them in a single layer on the rack.
- Season with pepper and salt and cook until very crisp; repeat with the rest of the kale.
- On a large cutting board or serving platter, pile crispy kale leaves.
- Heat a large grill pan over medium-high heat.

- Shake excess marinade off the chops then grill for 3 on each side, remove to a plate to rest while you grill the lemons cut side down.
- Serve with grilled lemon juice.
- Enjoy.

PEANUT CURRY WITH BROCCOLI AND TOFU

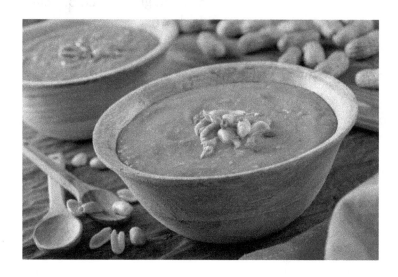

Peanut curry is made with a mixture of coconut milk and Thai curry paste for a creamy sauce, which is perfect with crispy tofu. This peanut butter curry is such an easy dinner you need to make for yourself. You can serve it with another grain of your choice if you prefer. It will be a dream for leftovers too.

PREP TIME: 15 mins
COOK TIME: 15 mins
TOTAL TIME: 30 mins
YIELD: 1 serving

NUTRITIONAL INFO

Calories: 413.91 cal | **Total fat:** 34.11 g | **Sugar:** 4.55 g | **Iron:** 5.17 mg | **Cholesterol:** 0 mg | **Carbohydrates:** 17.02 g | **Protein:** 15.78 g | **Fiber:** 32.95 g | **Calcium:** 158.91 mg | **Sodium:** 260.09 mg

INGREDIENTS

- 100 grams of Tofu
- 0.5 teaspoon of Soy Sauce
- 0.25 400grams tin of Coconut Milk
- 1 tablespoon of Peanut Butter
- 0.5 teaspoon of Red Curry Paste
- 0.25 Lime
- 0.25 teaspoon of Sugar
- 0.25 Red Pepper sliced
- 75 grams of tender-stem Broccoli
- 0.5 tablespoon of Cornflour
- Vegetable Oil
- 0.5 teaspoon of Ginger grated

DIRECTIONS

- Press the tofu for at least 10 minutes, then cut into cubes.
- In a large pot, heat a drizzle of oil and fry the tofu until browned on all sides.
- Set aside on a paper towel lined plate.
- Pour the coconut milk inside the pot and add the curry paste, peanut butter, soy sauce, juice of half the lime, and sugar.
- Heat until curry paste and peanut butter have melted into the sauce.
- Add the broccoli and pepper to the sauce.
- Cook for some minutes until softened slightly.
- Add the tofu back to the curry.
- Serve with rice and another half of a lime sliced into wedges.
- Enjoy.

STEAK SALAD

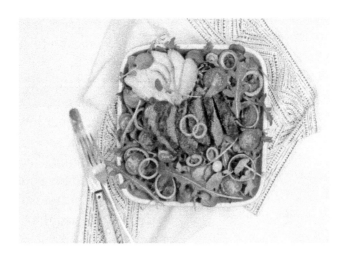

This is a Steak Salad with juicy slices and seasoned beef, which is on a bed of crunchy vegetables and colorful greens. It would be great if you can mix with a balsamic dressing.

This is made in a cast-iron skillet that cooks the meat to a perfect medium-rare.

PREP TIME: 35 mins
COOK TIME: 10 mins
TOTAL TIME: 45 mins
YIELD: 1 serving

NUTRITIONAL INFO

Calories: 615 cal | **Total fat:** 50 g | **Sugar:** 6 g | **Iron:** 3.6 mg | **Cholesterol:** 77 mg | **Carbohydrates:** 14 g | **Protein:** 29 g | **Fiber:** 6 g | **Calcium:** 163 mg | **Sodium:** 519 mg

INGREDIENTS

Balsamic Vinaigrette

- 0.06 cup (15 ml) of balsamic vinegar
- 0.5 teaspoons (2.5 ml) of Dijon mustard
- 0.13 teaspoon (0.5 g) of kosher salt
- 0.06 teaspoon of black pepper
- 0.13 cup (30 ml) of extra-virgin olive oil
- 0.25 teaspoon (1 g) of mayonnaise, optional

Steak Salad

- 0.13 cup (18 g) of thinly sliced cucumber
- 0.06 cup (8 g) of thinly sliced radish
- 0.06 cup (9.5 g) of diced red onion
- 0.5 tablespoon (7.5 ml) of olive oil
- 1 cups (18.75 g) of arugula, 1-inch pieces
- 0.25 medium avocado, sliced or diced

DIRECTIONS

- Whisk together mustard, vinegar, salt, mayonnaise and pepper in a medium bowl.
- Slowly drizzle in the olive oil.
- Whisk until it becomes a thickened emulsified dressing.
- Use paper towels to dry the surface of the steak.
- Season both sides with pepper and salt.
- Over high heat, heat a large cast-iron skillet until hot.
- Add the oil and add the steak once the oil is hot.
- Press it down into the pan.
- Cook for about 4 minutes until the surface is browned.
- Flip the steak and cook for about 3 to 5 minutes, until it reaches an internal temp of 120 to 125 degrees.
- Transfer the steak to a cutting board and rest for about 10 minutes.
- Slice the steak against the grain into 1/4 - inch thick pieces.
- Cut it smaller if you feel like.
- Mix together the romaine, arugula, and radicchio in a large serving bowl.

- 0.06 cup (10 g) of feta cheese
- 0.25 pound (113.5 g) of flank steak, or flat iron steak
- kosher salt, for seasoning
- 1 cups (35 g) of romaine lettuce
- 0.5 cups (15 g) of radicchio, 1-inch pieces
- 0.25 cup (40 g) of cherry tomatoes, cut in half

- Top salad with cucumber, tomatoes, onion, steak, radish, avocado, and feta cheese.
- Serve with balsamic vinaigrette.
- Enjoy.

LETTUCE WRAPS

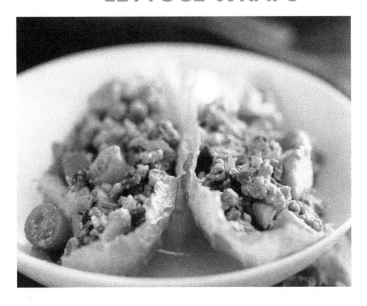

This Lettuce Wraps recipe is loaded with vegetables that are crunchy in a sweet, savory brown sauce. You can wrap with grounded shrimp or chicken.

You'll be wowed if you give this recipe a try. Lettuce wraps are so healthy, refreshing, crunchy, and delicious. They make the best light supper and taste way better than any lettuce wraps you have in mind. I'm sure of it!

PREP TIME: 20 mins
COOK TIME: 10 mins
TOTAL TIME: 30 mins
YIELD: 1 serving

NUTRITIONAL INFO

Calories: 114 cal | **Total fat:** 5 g | **Sugar:** 1 g | **Iron:** 1.2mg | **Cholesterol:** 95 mg | **Carbohydrates:** 3 g | **Protein:** 11 g | **Fiber:** 0 g | **Calcium:** 57mg | **Sodium:** 392 mg

INGREDIENTS

- Avocado oil
- 0.08 cup of chopped carrots (1 medium size carrot)
- 0.08 cup of chopped celery
- 0.5-0.63 whole water chestnuts, chopped
- 0.25 tablespoon of chopped garlic
- 0.13 large shallot, chopped
- 0.19 tablespoon of chopped ginger (3 thin slices)
- 0.06 pound of ground chicken breast
- 0.03 teaspoon of coarse salt
- 0.02 teaspoon of white pepper
- 0.06 pound of raw shrimp, diced and peeled with 1 teaspoon of arrowroot powder
Sauce (use 1 tablespoon at a time):
- 0.13 to 0.19 teaspoon of hot pepper sauce, optional
- 0.25 tablespoon of coconut Aminos

DIRECTIONS

- Get your ingredients ready and set it aside.
- Mix your shrimp with arrowroot if you'll be using.
- Add 3 tablespoons of oil in a well-heated large skillet.
- Sauté garlic, shallot, and ginger with a pinch of salt for about 10 seconds until fragrant.
- Add your ground chicken.
- Season with white pepper and salt.
- Break the meat into fine pieces. Sauté the meal for about 5 minutes until is cooked through. This time, your skillet should not be wet or watery.
- Add celery and carrots.
- Season with a pinch of salt and sauté for about 1 minute.
- Add shrimp and chestnuts.
- Sauté for another 1 minute if you'll be using it.
- Add stir-fry and sauce for 10 seconds.

- 0.06 tablespoon of almond butter

Serve and garnish:

- 0.13 whole large iceberg lettuce, leaves separated and tip edge trimmed (or 2 Boston lettuce)
- 0.38 tablespoon of lightly toasted pine nuts or chopped cashew nuts
- 0.13 bulb scallion, chopped
- Taste and make seasoning adjustments to your liking.
- Turn off the heat and garnish with scallions and pine nuts.
- Fill the lettuce cups with stir-fried ingredients.
- Serve hot and enjoy.

SAUTEED CHICORY GREENS

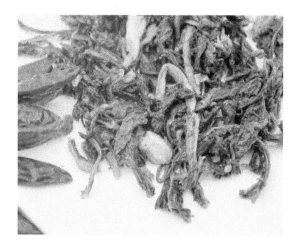

This Sautéed Chicory Greens is an easy and fresh meal you can prepare for dinner. It's just like cooked greens sautéed in garlic, olive oil, and a sprinkle of salt.

PREP TIME: 10 mins
COOK TIME: 2 mins
TOTAL TIME: 12 mins
YIELD: 1 serving

NUTRITIONAL INFO

Calories: 109 cal | **Total fat:** 9 g | **Sugar:** 0 g | **Iron:** 1.3 mg | **Cholesterol:** 0 mg | **Carbohydrates:** 5 g | **Protein:** 1 g | **Fiber:** 4 g | **Calcium:** 79 mg | **Sodium:** 421 mg

INGREDIENTS

- 0.33-0.67 cloves garlic, chopped
- 0.17 teaspoon of salt (2 1/2 grams)
- 0.33 bunch of chicory (1 pound /500-600 grams)
- 0.67-1 tablespoons of olive oil (26-39 grams)
- pinch of hot pepper flakes (if desired)

DIRECTIONS

- Wash the leaves and cut in half, cook in boiling water until tender but not mushy, drain well.
- Add garlic and olive oil in a medium frying pan, then add the salt, chicory, and hot pepper flakes.
- Toss gently and heat 2 minutes on medium heat.
- Serve immediately, with a squeeze of lemon if desired.
- Enjoy.

CAULIFLOWER FRIED RICE

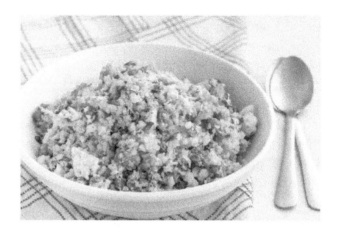

A beautiful recipe that can be made within 20 minutes and can be served as a side dish.

What gives this cauliflower fried rice an incredible flavor and satisfying texture is the combination of garlic, carrots, peas, green onions, scrambled eggs, soy sauce, and sesame oil.

PREP TIME: 5 mins
COOK TIME: 15 mins
TOTAL TIME: 20 mins
YIELD: 1 serving

NUTRITIONAL INFO

Calories: 163 cal | **Total fat:** 11 g | **Sugar:** 3 g | **Iron:** 1.5 mg | **Cholesterol:** 139 mg | **Carbohydrates:** 8 g | **Protein:** 8 g | **Fiber:** 2 g | **Calcium:** 44 mg | **Sodium:** 282 mg

INGREDIENTS

- 0.19 cup of peas fresh, canned or frozen and defrosted
- 0.5 tablespoons of soy sauce
- 0.06 teaspoon of sesame oil
- 0.5 cloves of garlic minced
- 0.19 cup of carrots (1/4-inch dice)
- 0.5 tablespoons of green onion thinly sliced
- 0.25 large head of cauliflower
- 0.5 tablespoons of vegetable oil divided
- 0.75 large eggs beaten

DIRECTIONS

- Remove the outer leaves of the cauliflower using a knife.
- Cut off the cauliflower florets from the stem.
- Cut florets into 1-inch sized pieces.
- In a food processor, add florets and pulse until small pieces form, scraping the sides of the bowl as needed.
- In the food processor, work in batches for larger heads of cauliflower.
- Remove from the food processor or blender if larger pieces of cauliflower do not get processed.
- Cut into smaller florets, then process after removing the cut cauliflower rice from the food processor.
- Chop cauliflower florets into small rice-sized pieces with a knife, processed or grated with a blender.
- Over medium-high heat, heat a large skillet or a wok.
- Add the minced garlic once hot and stir fry until fragrant but not browned, for about 30 seconds.

- Add the carrots and cook until tender, for about 2 minutes.
- Add the peas and cook for a minute.
- Add the cauliflower and stir to combine.
- Spread the cauliflower mixture out in the pan and allow to cook for about 2 minutes without stirring.
- Mix the rice and stir fry for about 5 minutes until the cauliflower rice is tender.
- Add the sesame oil and soy sauce, stirring to combine.
- Taste the rice and add more salt, soy sauce, and pepper as needed.
- Reduce heat to medium and make a big well in the center of the pan. Allow it to warm.
- Add n the eggs once hot.
- Stir to cook and break the eggs into small scrambled pieces (use quick stir motion).
- Stir together with the cauliflower rice once cooked.
- Garnish cauliflower rice with sliced green onions.
- Serve hot and enjoy.

SPICY MEATBALLS

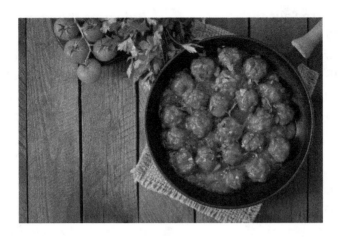

Spicy meatballs are boldly flavored with cumin, paprika, garlic, and cayenne.

The sauce used for this recipe is incredible and can be served with cauliflower rice or meatballs over rice.

PREP TIME: 15 mins
COOK TIME: 30 mins
TOTAL TIME: 45 mins
YIELD: 1 serving

NUTRITIONAL INFO

Calories: 315 cal | **Total fat:** 20 g | **Sugar:** 0 g | **Iron:** 0 mg | **Cholesterol:** 0 mg | **Carbohydrates:** 9 g | **Protein:** 22 g | **Fiber:** 3 g | **Calcium:** 0 mg | **Sodium:** 650 mg

INGREDIENTS

Tomato Sauce:
- 0.25 teaspoon of sweet paprika
- 0.25 teaspoon of ground cumin
- 0.06 teaspoon of cayenne pepper
- 0.25 tablespoon of olive oil
- 0.25 tablespoon of minced garlic
- 0.25 teaspoon of Diamond Crystal kosher salt
- 6.5 ounces of Pomi chopped tomatoes, or two 15 ounces cans of diced tomatoes, undrained

Meatballs:
- 0.25 teaspoon of ground cumin
- 0.25 teaspoon of ground coriander
- 0.13 teaspoon of ground cinnamon
- 0.06 teaspoon of cayenne pepper
- 0.25 pound of 85% lean ground beef
- 0.25 teaspoon of Diamond Crystal kosher salt

DIRECTIONS

Preparing the tomato sauce:
- In heavy saucepan, heat the olive oil over medium heat for about 3 minutes.
- Add the garlic and cook for about 1 minute.
- Add the spices and cook, stirring for 30 seconds.
- Add the chopped tomatoes.
- Bring to boil and lower heat to medium-low, then simmer, covered for about 10 minutes.

Preparing the meatballs:
- Use your hands to mix the spices and meat in a medium bowl.
- Divide into 24 equal portions and shape into small 1 inch meatballs.
- Add the meatballs to the tomato sauce.
- Turn heat to medium-high and bring to a boil, then lower heat back to medium-low.
- Cover, simmer for about 30 minutes.
- Sprinkle with the cilantro.
- Serve and enjoy.

- 0.25 teaspoon of onion powder
- 0.25 teaspoon of sweet paprika

Garnish:

- 0.5 tablespoons of finely chopped fresh cilantro

PUMPKIN PASTA

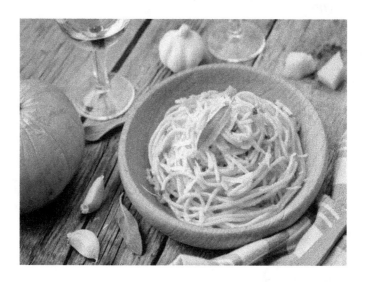

This Pumpkin Pasta is a portion of homemade pasta, looking so fluffy and fresh. This pumpkin is more of a hint, super flavorful pasta, and way to add some color to your meal.

You don't need many ingredients for this pasta. All you need is egg, flour, salt, water, and pumpkin puree. That's so easy!

PREP TIME: 43 mins
COOK TIME: 2 mins
TOTAL TIME: 45 mins
YIELD: 1 serving

NUTRITIONAL INFO

Calories: 279 cal | **Total fat:** 4 g | **Sugar:** 0.8 g | **Iron:** 0 mg | **Cholesterol:** 0 mg | **Carbohydrates:** 48 g | **Protein:** 11 g | **Fiber:** 2 g | **Calcium:** 0 mg | **Sodium:** 165 mg

INGREDIENTS

- 2 egg yolks
- 3 tablespoons of pumpkin puree
- Water
- 2 cups of unbleached all-purpose flour
- 1/4 teaspoon of sea salt
- 1 large egg

DIRECTIONS

- Add salt and flour into a food processor and pulse.
- Add in egg yolks, whole egg, and pumpkin puree.
- Pulse until it's well combined.
- Drizzle in water until a dough forms.
- Transfer to a very lightly floured surface.
- Sprinkle the top with a little flour.
- Cover with plastic wrap and set it aside for about 30 minutes.
- Bring a large pot of water to a boil and salt generously until it's rested.
- Cut the pasta into thirds and start rolling out into a loose rectangle.
- Sprinkle on only as much flour as it takes to keep it from sticking.
- More flour and less flavorful, tender pasta.
- The pasta will want to stick to the rolling pin, so what you have to do is use one hand to hold it down while you use the other to roll
- Cut dough into any shape you want. Cover with plastic wrap till it's ready to cook.
- Add pasta to boiling water and stir together.
- Drain and transfer into a serving plate.
- Top with Parmesan cheese and pesto.
- Toss with your favorite tomato sauce.
- Serve and enjoy.

CHORIZO POTATOES

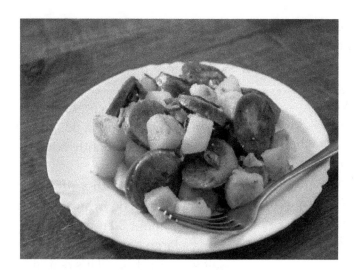

Do you know that chorizo potatoes can be made with just 3 to 4 ingredients? With these natural ingredients, you can get your meal ready for dinner with simple huevos rancheros, which will make you fall in love.

The potatoes are pan-fried, creating a caramelized roasted flavor on the potatoes.

PREP TIME: 5 mins
COOK TIME: 30 mins
TOTAL TIME: 35 mins
YIELD: 1 serving

NUTRITIONAL INFO

Calories: 241 cal | **Total fat:** 6 g | **Sugar:** 2 g | **Iron:** 0 mg | **Cholesterol:** 12 mg | **Carbohydrates:** 40 g | **Protein:** 8 g | **Fiber:** 4 g | **Calcium:** 0 mg | **Sodium:** 243 mg

INGREDIENTS

- 3 ounces of beef Chorizo
- 1 clove garlic
- 2.5 pounds of Yukon Gold potatoes chopped small
- Salt and pepper to taste

DIRECTIONS

- Over medium heat add potatoes and a drizzle of olive oil in a skillet.
- Place a lid on the pan.
- Cook, stirring occasionally until the potatoes are tender and roasted, for about 10 minutes.
- Remove the lid, adding some oil if needed, and continue to cook the potatoes, increasing the heat to medium-high if needed until browned.
- Add the garlic and chorizo in another pan over medium heat.
- Place a splatter screen over the pan as it can be very messy.
- Cook, stirring occasionally for 6 mins.
- Strain any excess liquid from the chorizo using a mesh strainer.
- Add the chorizo mixture to the potatoes.
- Cook, stirring as needed until everything is evenly coated.
- Sprinkle with pepper and a little salt to taste.
- Serve immediately and enjoy.

BASIL WITH TOMATO SAUCE

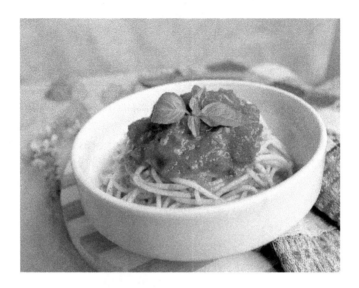

This kind of recipe saves both money and time. With this recipe, you'll be having a tasty sauce perfectly okay with pasta, fish, or meat.

You need to give it a try today!

PREP TIME: 5 mins
COOK TIME: 10 mins
TOTAL TIME: 15 mins
YIELD: 1 serving

NUTRITIONAL INFO

Calories: 52 cal | **Total fat:** 3 g | **Sugar:** 4 g | **Iron:** 0 mg | **Cholesterol:** 12 mg | **Carbohydrates:** 5 g | **Protein:** 2 g | **Fiber:** 1 g | **Calcium:** 0 mg | **Sodium:** 0 mg

INGREDIENTS

- 1 tablespoon of tomato purée
- 1 teaspoon of sugar
- 1 tablespoon of olive oil
- 1 garlic clove, crushed
- 400grams can of chopped tomatoes
- 1 teaspoon of vegetable stock powder or 1/2 crumbled stock cube
- few basil leaves

DIRECTIONS

- In a pan, heat 1 tablespoon of olive oil.
- Add 1 crushed garlic clove and gently fry for a minute.
- Tip in 400grams of chopped tomatoes, 1/2 crumbled stock cube or 1 tablespoon of vegetable stock powder, 1 tablespoon of tomato puree and 1 teaspoon of sugar, then bring it to boil.
- Reduce the heat and then simmer uncovered for about 5 minutes, stirring occasionally.
- Tear some basil leaves and then stir into the sauce.
- Serve and enjoy.

CHORIZO WITH RIGATONI PASTA

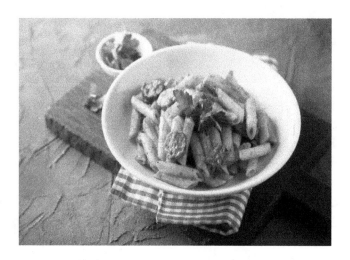

Chorizo with Rigatoni Pasta is great for a dinner meal. You can make it vegetarian and makes it taste great!

This recipe would need more chorizo because I don't think it's excellent without chorizo. Chorizo makes this recipe fancy and delicious.

PREP TIME: 25 mins
COOK TIME: 25 mins
TOTAL TIME: 50 mins
YIELD: 1 serving

NUTRITIONAL INFO

Calories: 574.5 cal | **Total fat:** 30.3 g | **Sugar:** 6.9 g | **Iron:** 3.9 mg | **Cholesterol:** 70.2 mg | **Carbohydrates:** 50.1 g | **Protein:** 25.3 g | **Fiber:** 2.9 g

INGREDIENTS

- 1/8 (16 ounce) package of rigatoni pasta
- 1/4 cup of whole milk
- 1/8 (14.5 ounce) can of diced tomatoes, undrained
- 1/8 teaspoon of salt
- 1/8 teaspoon of pepper
- 3/4 teaspoon of butter
- 1/4 clove garlic, minced
- 2 ounces of chorizo sausage links, sliced
- 3/4 teaspoon of butter
- 3/4 teaspoon of flour
- 1-1/2 teaspoons of Parmesan cheese, grated
- 1/8 onion, diced
- 1/8 green bell pepper, diced

DIRECTIONS

- Bring a large pot of salted water to a boil.
- Add rigatoni and cook for about 8 minutes, until al dente. Drain it.
- In a large skillet, melt 1 tablespoon of butter over medium heat.
- Stir in the onion, garlic, and bell pepper.
- Cook and stir until the onion has turned translucent and softened, for about 5 minutes.
- Add chorizo slices and cook until the chorizo is no longer pink in the center, for about 10 minutes.
- In a saucepan, melt the remaining 2 tablespoons of butter over medium heat.
- Whisk in the flour and cook for about 5 minutes, stirring constantly.
- Slowly whisk in the milk. Over medium-high heat, bring it to a simmer.
- Add the salt, diced tomatoes, and pepper, then reduce the heat to medium-low and simmer for about 10 minutes to smooth and thicken the sauce.
- Stir the cooked chorizo into the sauce with the drained rigatoni pasta.
- Stir and sprinkle with Parmesan cheese to serve. Serve and enjoy.

KALE SUPER SALAD

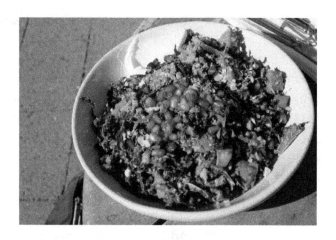

Kale salad is a super salad that is gorgeous and perfect. It's full of nutrients and amazing flavor. By the way, this recipe is for one.

This is the kind of recipe that will bring balance to your dinner diet. You will crave it more most, especially if you happen to be a Kale lover!

PREP TIME: 20 mins
COOK TIME: 20 mins
TOTAL TIME: 40 mins
YIELD: 1 serving

NUTRITIONAL INFO

Calories: 321 cal | **Total fat:** 14 g | **Sugar:** 19 g | **Iron:** 3.2 mg | **Cholesterol:** 18 mg | **Carbohydrates:** 39 g | **Protein:** 15 g | **Fiber:** 7 g | **Calcium:** 192 mg | **Sodium:** 398 mg

INGREDIENTS

Dressing:

- 0.2 whole lemon juice and zested
- 0.1 teaspoon of salt
- 0.05 teaspoon of pepper
- 0.4+0.2 tablespoons of olive oil
- 1 shallots
- 0.3 cups of chopped dried cranberries
- 0.8 tablespoons of red wine vinegar
- 0.2 tablespoon of honey

Salad Mix:

- 0.6 apples you can use chopped Honey-crisp
- 0.2 cup of pistachios
- 0.3 cups of bacon bite you can use fresh bacon, cook and roughly chopped
- 2.4 cups of kale chopped
- 4.8 Brussels sprouts thinly sliced/shredded
- 0.6 small heads of broccoli finely chopped
- 0.2 pomegranate use all the seeds

Optional Topping:

- 1.6 ounces crumbled of goat cheese

DIRECTIONS

For the dressing:

- In a large sauté pan, add 2 tablespoons of olive oil over medium-high heat.
- Add finely sliced shallot and cook until tender, for about 5 minutes.
- Remove from the heat, set it aside till you're ready to mix salad.
- Add garlic and sauté for about 2 minutes.
- Then add red wine vinegar, chopped cranberries, honey, lemon juice, zest, and the rest tablespoon of olive oil.
- Stir to combine and season with pepper and salt.
- Remove from heat and set it aside.

For the salad:

- In a large salad bowl, add Brussels sprouts, kale, broccoli, apples, bacon, pomegranate seeds, and pistachios. Toss to combine.
- Add goat cheese and dressing if you feel like and toss to combine.
- Serve immediately and enjoy.

SURF AND TURF

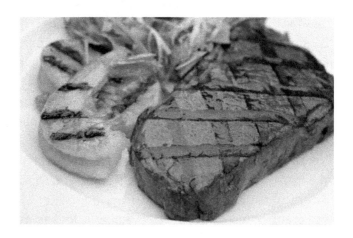

Surf and Turf is a simple way to make a special dinner for yourself. In this recipe, you probably have most of the ingredients in your pantry.

Yeah, it would be best if you had everything already. Serve alongside steaks with your favorite side dishes. This recipe is beyond delicious, and if you follow correctly like the instructions, it would be enjoyable. I promise!

PREP TIME: 15 mins
COOK TIME: 15 mins
TOTAL TIME: 30 mins
YIELD: 1 serving

NUTRITIONAL INFO

Calories: 443.9 cal | **Total fat:** 35.2 g | **Sugar:** 0 g | **Iron:** 4.2 mg | **Cholesterol:** 165.9 mg | **Carbohydrates:** 2.9 g | **Protein:** 26.9 g | **Fiber:** 0.3 g | **Calcium:** 47.5 mg | **Sodium:** 925.8 mg

INGREDIENTS

- 1/2 teaspoon of lemon juice
- 1/2 teaspoon of dried parsley
- 1 teaspoon of olive oil
- 1-1/2 teaspoons of melted butter
- 1-1/2 teaspoons of finely minced onion
- 1/8 teaspoon of freshly ground black pepper
- 6 medium shrimp, peeled and deveined
- 1 (4 ounce) filet mignon steaks
- 1 teaspoon of olive oil
- 1/2 teaspoon of steak seasoning
- 1-1/2 teaspoons of white wine
- 1/2 teaspoon of Worcestershire sauce
- 1/2 teaspoon of seafood seasoning (such as Old Bay®)
- 1/2 clove garlic, minced

DIRECTIONS

- Whisk butter, 1 tablespoon of olive oil, wine, onion, lemon juice, Worcestershire sauce, garlic, seafood seasoning, and black pepper together in a bowl.
- Add shrimp and toss to coat evenly.
- Cover the bowl with plastic wrap.
- Refrigerate for flavors to blend for about 15 minutes.
- Preheat an outdoor grill to medium-high heat.
- Oil the grate slightly.
- Coat steaks with 2 tablespoons of olive oil.
- Sprinkle with steak seasoning.
- Cook steaks until they begin to firm and reach their desired doneness, for about 5 minutes per side.
- Transfer steaks into a platter and tent loosely with a piece of aluminum foil.
- Remove shrimp from marinade.
- Grill until they are bright pink on the outside, for about 2 minutes per side or until meat.

- Serve and enjoy.

GARLIC LEMON SCALLOPS

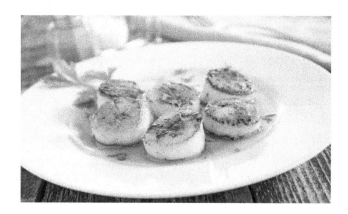

This is scallops sautéed in garlic and butter will melt in your mouth.

If you make this dinner recipe, you'll pleasantly be surprised with the results. It's a recipe that is so simple and delicious. Just follow exactly, and do not change anything.

PREP TIME: 10 mins
COOK TIME: 10 mins
TOTAL TIME: 20 mins
YIELD: 1 serving

NUTRITIONAL INFO

Calories: 408 cal | **Total fat:** 24.4 g | **Sugar:** 0.2 g | **Iron:** 3.6 mg | **Cholesterol:** 154.2 mg | **Carbohydrates:** 8.9 g | **Protein:** 38.5 g | **Fiber:** 0.1 g | **Calcium:** 71.5 mg | **Sodium:** 987.9 mg

INGREDIENTS

- 5 ounces of large sea scallops
- 1/8 teaspoon of salt
- 1/8 teaspoon of pepper
- 2 tablespoons of butter
- 1-1/2 teaspoons of minced garlic
- 1 teaspoon of fresh lemon juice

DIRECTIONS

- In a large skillet, melt butter over medium-high heat.
- Stir in garlic and cook for some seconds until fragrant.
- Add scallops and cook for some minutes one side, then turn over and go-ahead with the cooking till opaque and firm.
- Remove scallops to a platter and then whisk pepper, salt, and lemon juice into butter.
- Pour sauce over scallops to serve.
- Serve and enjoy.

TERIYAKI TEMPEH

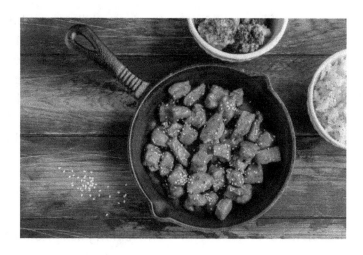

Teriyaki Tempeh makes a perfect protein addition to any meal. Okay?

So you don't have to worry at all. This is because Tempeh contains more protein and fiber than tofu. After all, it is less processed. It's a good source of magnesium, potassium, iron, and vitamin B6.

PREP TIME: 20 mins
COOK TIME: 20 mins
TOTAL TIME: 40 mins
YIELD: 1 serving

NUTRITIONAL INFO

Calories: 211 cal | **Total fat:** 11 g | **Sugar:** 0 g | **Iron:** 4.9 mg | **Cholesterol:** 0 mg | **Carbohydrates:** 14 g | **Protein:** 14 g | **Fiber:** 2 g | **Calcium:** 70 mg | **Sodium:** 0 mg

INGREDIENTS

- 0.25 tablespoon of olive or coconut oil
- 0.25 (8 ounces) package of organic tempeh

Tempeh Marinade:

- 0.13 teaspoon of garlic powder
- 0.06 teaspoon of onion powder
- 0.75 tablespoon of veggie broth
- 0.25 tablespoon of tamari (or soy sauce)

Teriyaki Sauce:

- 0.25 teaspoon of rice wine or apple cider vinegar
- 0.13 teaspoon of garlic powder
- 0.13 teaspoon of corn starch
- 1 tablespoon of tamari (or soy sauce)
- 0.25 teaspoon of sesame or olive oil
- 0.5 tablespoon of maple syrup
- 0.25 teaspoon of sriracha (or hot sauce)
- 0.06 teaspoon of liquid smoke (optional but tasty)

DIRECTIONS

- In a steamer basket, cut tempeh into triangles or maybe, squares for about 10 minutes.
- Add all of the ingredients for the marinade into the bowl and then whisk together.
- Place tempeh into the dish and pour marinade over it.
- Marinate for about 20 minutes.
- In a pan, place coconut or olive oil and sear the tempeh for about 3 to 5 minutes on each side until crispy.
- In a large bowl, mix the teriyaki sauce ingredients.
- Add tempeh to teriyaki sauce once tempeh is cooked, covering the tempeh.
- Take the tempeh out of the sauce and add it back to the pan.
- Heat tempeh again for about 30 seconds on each side to caramelize the sauce on the tempeh.
- Turn off the heat and pour the rest of the sauce over the tempeh in the pan.

Toppings:
- Scallions
- Sesame seeds

- Leave it for 1 minute to the rest of the sauce. This will make it thicken a little bit.
- Serve and top with scallions and sesame if you feel like.
- Enjoy.

OKONOMIYAKI

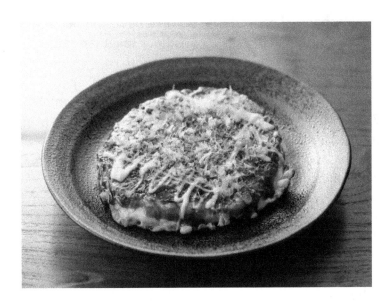

The word Okonomi means 'what you like,' and yaki means 'grilled.' Okonomiyaki is from Japanese. It's a Japanese pancake that's stuffed with yummy goodness.

You can feel free to add any other meats or vegetables. Just have fun playing with the ingredients.

PREP TIME: 10 mins
COOK TIME: 10 mins
TOTAL TIME: 20 mins
YIELD: 1 serving

NUTRITIONAL INFO

Calories: 328.8 cal | **Total fat:** 15.1 g | **Sugar:** 0 g | **Iron:** 3.2 mg | **Cholesterol:** 128 mg | **Carbohydrates:** 33.3 g | **Protein:** 15.7 g | **Fiber:** 3.5 g | **Calcium:** 125.1 mg | **Sodium:** 879.1 mg

INGREDIENTS

- 1 tablespoon of cooked shrimp (optional)
- 2-1/2 teaspoons of shredded cheese (optional)
- 7-1/2 cups of tenkasu (tempura pearls)
- 3/4 teaspoon of vegetable oil, or to taste1/41/4 cup of all-purpose flour
- 2 tablespoons and 2 teaspoons of water
- 1 cup of chopped cabbage
- 1-1/2 strips of cooked bacon, crumbled
- 1/2 eggs
- 1/4 sausage, diced, or more to taste (optional)
- 2 tablespoons of chopped green onions
  Toppings:
- 1 tablespoon of panko bread crumbs, or to taste
- 1 teaspoon of mayonnaise, or to taste
- 2 tablespoons of soy sauce
- 1 tablespoon of ketchup
- 1 teaspoon of white vinegar

DIRECTIONS

- In a bowl, mix water and flour together until smooth.
- Stir in bacon, eggs, cabbage, green onions, sausage, shrimp, tenkasu, and cheese.
- Preheat a griddle to 400 degrees F.
- Coat with oil and pour in flour mixture into the shape of a pancake.
- Cook for about 6 minutes per side until golden brown.
- Transfer to a serving plate.
- Mix ketchup, soy sauce, and vinegar together in a small bowl to make your okonomiyaki sauce.
- Drizzle over pancake.
- Garnish with mayonnaise and panko.
- Serve and enjoy.

KEEMA CURRY

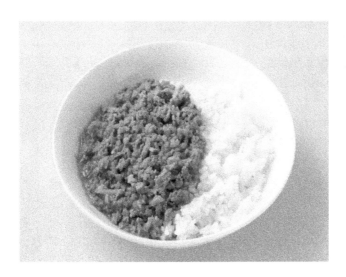

Keema curry is from India. It's an Indian curry dish made of minced vegetables and ground meat (lamb). This kind of curry has been adapted to Japanese taste.

I'm sure you will add this recipe to your favorite dish. It's so easy to make and not only tastes good.

PREP TIME: 10 mins
COOK TIME: 20 mins
TOTAL TIME: 30 mins
YIELD: 1 serving

NUTRITIONAL INFO

Calories: 800.3 cal | **Total fat:** 30.2 g | **Sugar:** 0 g | **Iron:** 9 mg | **Cholesterol:** 362 mg | **Carbohydrates:** 79.3 g | **Protein:** 132.7 g | **Fiber:** 13.2 g | **Calcium:** 112 mg | **Sodium:** 2301 mg

INGREDIENTS

- 1/4 teaspoon of kosher/sea salt
- freshly ground black pepper
- 1 onion (7 ounces or 200 grams)
- 1 teaspoon of curry powder
- 1 tablespoon of unsalted butter
- 2 cubes Japanese curry roux
- 1 tablespoon of ketchup
- 1 tablespoon of Tonkatsu sauce
- 1 stalk celery (2 ounces or 57 grams)
- 1/2 carrot (3.5 ounces or 100 grams)
- 6 shiitake mushrooms (soak in if you use dried shiitake mushrooms, soak in 1 cup of water for about 15 mins and squeeze the water out and then use this Shiitake Dashi in place of water.

DIRECTIONS

- Gather all of the ingredients.
- Firstly, prepare steamed rice if you don't have any.
- Mince the celery, onion, shiitake mushrooms, and carrot.
- Heat oil over medium heat in a large skillet.
- Sauté the onion until translucent.
- Add ground pork and cook until no longer pink.
- Season with pepper and salt.
- Add carrots, shiitake mushrooms, and celery and then mix well with the remaining ingredients.
- Add water and chicken stock.
- Add extra water if necessary so the liquid is just enough to cover the ingredients.
- Add the curry powder and mix well.
- Cover and bring to a boil.
- Skim off the foam and scum on the surface with a fine mesh skimmer.
- Reduce the heat to medium-low heat and cook covered for about 5 minutes, until the carrot is tender.
- Add butter and curry roux and mix well.

196

- 1 tablespoon of neutral-flavored oil (canola, vegetable, canola)
- 1 pound of ground pork (454 g; for vegan/vegetarian, use mushrooms, eggplant, zucchini, etc)
- 1 cup of chicken broth
- 1/2 cup of water (or more)

Toppings (optional)
- fried eggs

- Add tonkatsu sauce and ketchup
- Mix well and simmer without covering for 2 minutes.
- Add a small amount of water if the sauce is too thick.
- Serve your curry over steamed rice if you want. Enjoy.

BEEF BURRITO

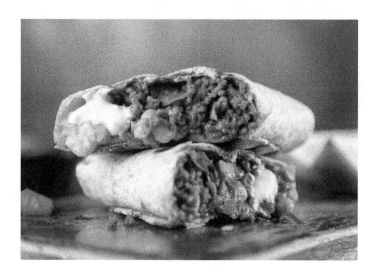

This is spicy beef burritos that contain various seasonings and peppers on top of refried beans. You can top off with sour cream, lettuce, cheese, and lastly, wrap up in a softshell.

You'll go crazy over these burritos. Do not change anything and make the recipe accurately as called for. It's so perfect and incredibly yummy for dinner!

PREP TIME: 30 mins
COOK TIME: 20 mins
TOTAL TIME: 50 mins
YIELD: 1 serving

NUTRITIONAL INFO
Calories: 120 cal | **Total fat:** 38.9 g | **Sugar:** 6.5 g | **Iron:** 9 mg | **Cholesterol:** 25 mg | **Carbohydrates:** 50.9 g | **Protein:** 34 g | **Fiber:** 8.5 g | **Calcium:** 400 mg | **Sodium:** 600 mg

INGREDIENTS

- 1/8 (1 ounce) package of burrito seasoning
- 1/8 (14 ounce) can of refried beans
- 1 (10 inch) flour tortillas
- 1/8 (10 ounce) bag of shredded lettuce
- 1/8 (8 ounce) container of sour cream
- 3/4 teaspoon of hot sauce
- 1/8 teaspoon of ground cayenne pepper
- 2-1/2 ounces of ground beef
- 1 ounce of sliced jalapeno peppers
- 1/8 tomato, diced
- 1/8 (4 ounces) can of chopped green chile peppers
- 1/8 green bell pepper, diced
- 1/8 red bell pepper, diced
- 1/8 onion, diced
- 1/8 (8 ounce) package of shredded sharp Cheddar cheese

DIRECTIONS

- In a large bowl, mix tomato, jalapeno peppers, green bell pepper, green chili peppers, onion, red bell pepper, hot sauce, and cayenne pepper.
- In a large skillet, cook beef over medium-high heat.
- Stirring to break up clumps, for about 5 mins.
- Drain excess grease and add the jalapeno pepper mixture with burrito seasoning.
- Cook and covered, stirring occasionally for about 10 minutes until flavors combine.
- In a saucepan over medium low heat, pour your re-fried beans.
- Cook and stir until heated through for about 5 minutes.
- In the microwave, warm each tortilla for about 15 seconds, until soft.
- Spread a layer of re-fried beans on top.
- Divide beef mixture among the tortilla.
- Top with sour cream, lettuce, and cheddar cheese.
- Fold in opposing edges of each tortilla. Roll up into a burrito.
- Serve and enjoy.

NASI GORENG

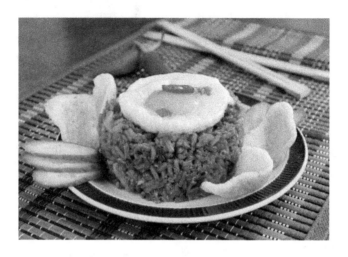

I love the word 'Nasi Goreng.' This recipe is a recipe from Indonesia. It's Indonesia's version of fried rice, and it gets a sweet-savory from shrimp paste.

Terasi will be used in this recipe. It provides both your senses and your kitchen. You can feel free to substitute for another shrimp paste (or omit) if you can't find it easily.

PREP TIME: 20 mins
COOK TIME: 20 mins
TOTAL TIME: 40 mins
YIELD: 1 serving

NUTRITIONAL INFO

Calories: 640 cal | **Total fat:** 0 g | **Sugar:** 6.5 g | **Iron:** 0 mg | **Cholesterol:** 23 mg | **Carbohydrates:** 576 g | **Protein:** 48 g | **Fiber:** 32 g | **Calcium:** 1 mg | **Sodium:** 0 mg

INGREDIENTS

For the Spice Paste:
- 1/2 teaspoon of terasi (Indonesian shrimp paste), optional
- 2 small shallots (2 ounces; 55g), roughly chopped
- 3 medium cloves garlic
- 1 large fresh green chili, such as Fresno or Holland, stemmed and seeded, or 1 teaspoon of sambal oelek, such as Huy Fong

For the Nasi Goreng:
- 2 tablespoons (30ml) of neutral oil, such as canola or sunflower oil
- 2 tablespoons (30ml) of kecap manis, plus more for drizzling
- 2 teaspoons (10ml) of soy sauce
- Kosher salt
- Ground white pepper
- 4 cups of cold cooked jasmine rice (21 ounces; 600g)

To Serve:
- 2 fried eggs, cooked sunny-side-up or over easy

DIRECTIONS

For the Spice Paste:
- Add half of the shallots into a mortar and grind with the pestle till coarse puree forms.
- Add garlic, the remaining shallots, terasi, and chili, grinding with the pestle till each of the ingredients are mostly incorporated just before adding the next.
- In a food processor, combine all spice paste ingredients until they form a paste.

For the Nasi Goreng:
- Transfer rice to a bowl and break the rice up with your hands
- In a large skillet, heat oil over high heat until shimmering.
- Add spice paste and cook, stirring constantly and scraping the bottom of the pan to prevent the paste from burning until a smell permeates your kitchen for about 2 minutes and paste turns a little darker.
- Reduce the heat to medium if the paste appears to be browning

- Sliced cucumbers (optional)
- Sliced tomatoes (optional)
- Fried shallots (optional)

- too quickly.
- Add rice to your skillet and stir to coat with the spice paste.
- Add rice to your skillet and stir to coat with the spice paste.
- Add soy sauce and kecap manis.
- Stir and cook until rice is hot throughout and evenly colored.
- Season with white pepper and salt.
- Garnish with tomato and cucumber slices and shower with fried shallots if you want.
- Serve immediately and enjoy.

BEEF RENDANG

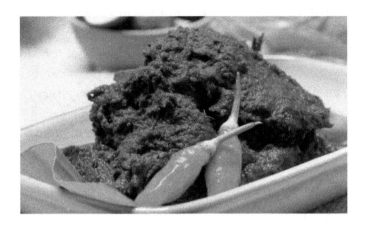

Congratulations to you if you choose to try this recipe. Rendang is the world's most delicious food from Indonesia.

This Beef rendang is served on special occasions during festive seasons and to honor guests. It's a delicious dish from Indonesia prepared with spices and a myriad of herbs until all liquids have absorbed by the meat entirely for a few hours.

It is best eaten/served with steamed rice.

PREP TIME: 30 mins
COOK TIME: 3 hours
TOTAL TIME: 3 hours 30 mins
YIELD: 1 serving

NUTRITIONAL INFO

Calories: 1533 cal | **Total fat:** 90 g | **Sugar:** 83 g | **Iron:** 0 mg | **Cholesterol:** 187 mg | **Carbohydrates:** 125 g | **Protein:** 64 g | **Fiber:** 9 g | **Calcium:** 0 mg | **Sodium:** 1863 mg

INGREDIENTS

- 600 ml of coconut cream
- 100 ml of vegetable oil
- 1 kg beef
- **Blending:**
- 4 candlenuts
- 12 cloves of chopped garlic
- 300 grams of red chili, (Serrano chili/pepper)
- 250 grams of onions
- 1 tablespoon of salt
- 1 teaspoon of sugar
- 4 green cardamom pods
- 11/2 teaspoon of cumin seeds
- 10 cloves
- 50 grams of ginger
- 50 grams of galangal
- 25 grams of ground turmeric, or 50grams of fresh turmeric
- 1 1/2 teaspoon of ground coriander
- **Spices and seasonings:**
- 1 piece of asam keping
- 2 turmeric leaves, tied up

DIRECTIONS

- Cut the beef into 4 centimeter squares.
- Don't cut the beef too small because the meat can bread into small pieces when cooking.
- Blend all of the blending ingredients and set it aside.
- Remove the outer sheath of the lemongrass and green section.
- Use just the white portion.
- Bash them so the lemongrass to ensure the release of the flavor.
- In a skillet, heat up the vegetable oil.
- Sauté the spices over low heat until aromatic.
- Add the turmeric leaves, coconut cream, asam keping, kaffir lime leaves, and lemongrass into the skillet.
- Add the beef and cook beef over medium heat.
- Bring the coconut milk to a boil.
- Continue simmering over low heat once it is boiled.
- Add water from time to time when the stem is about to dry.

- 4 stalks of bashed lemongrass
- 3 pieces of kaffir lime leaves

- Cook until the beef absorbs the flavor of the spices thoroughly and the color turns to dark brown. about 3 hours.
- Serve with bread or rice.
- Enjoy.

FRIED FISH VEGETABLE

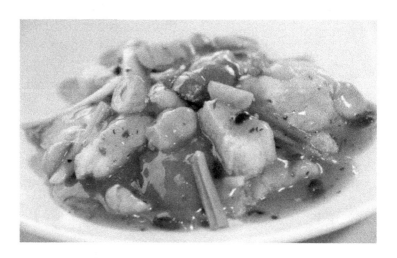

Fried Fish Vegetables is the kind of meal that can be prepared within 25 minutes. It holds their shape during stir-frying, such as whitefish or cod. They work best for this recipe as well.

PREP TIME: 10 mins
COOK TIME: 0 mins
TOTAL TIME: 25 mins
YIELD: 1 serving

NUTRITIONAL INFO

Calories: 250 cal | Total fat: 11 g | Sugar: 3 g | Iron: 0 mg | Cholesterol: 65 mg | Carbohydrates: 11 g | Protein: 24 g | Fiber: 4 g | Calcium: 0 mg | Sodium: 460 mg

INGREDIENTS

- 1 tablespoon of oyster sauce
- 1 teaspoon of granulated sugar
- 4 teaspoons of water
- 1 pound of fish fillets, sliced into 1/2-inch cubes
- 2 tablespoons of light soy sauce
- 1 tablespoon of Chinese rice wine
- 1/2 teaspoon of sesame oil
- 8 ounces of sliced mushrooms
- 1/4 teaspoon of salt
- 1/2 medium yellow bell pepper, chopped and seeded
- 1/2 medium red bell pepper, chopped and seeded
- 1/2 medium green bell pepper, chopped and seeded
- 1 cup of chopped scallions
- 3 teaspoons of cornstarch, divided
- 1/8 cup of chicken broth

DIRECTIONS

- In a medium bowl, place fish cubes and add soy sauce, sesame oil, rice wine, and 2 tablespoons of cornstarch. Marinate for about 15 minutes.
- Combine oyster sauce, chicken broth, and sugar in a bowl.
- Dissolve 1 teaspoon of cornstarch into 4 teaspoons of water in a separate small bowl. Set it aside.
- Heat a medium skillet over medium-high heat until it's nearly smoking.
- Add 2 tablespoons of oil. Add half the ginger when oil is hot and stir fry for about 10 seconds.
- Add fish cubes and stir fry until they start to brown, for about 2 minutes.
- Remove fish and drain on paper towels or in a colander.
- Heat 1 tablespoon of oil in the skillet.
- Add the remainder of ginger when oil is hot.
- Stir-fry and then add mushrooms.

- 3 tablespoons of peanut oil, divided
- 2 teaspoons of minced ginger, divided

- Stir-fry for about 1 minute, sprinkling with salt.
- Add bell pepper and stir-fry for an extra minute.
- Splash vegetables with 1 to 2 tablespoons of water when they start to dry out.
- Push vegetables to the sides of the pan.
- Add chicken broth mixture and then boil it.
- Stir water and cornstarch and add into the sauce, stirring quickly to thicken.
- Add fish back into the pan once the sauce has thick-end.
- Stir-fry for an extra minute to combine ingredients.
- Top with scallions.
- Serve and enjoy.

FISH FINGERS

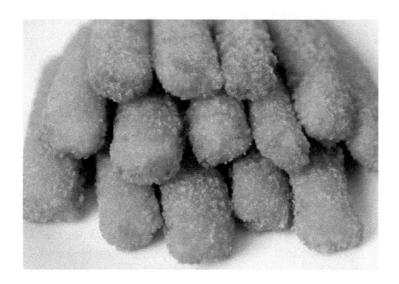

Fish Fingers are perfectly crunchy and golden. Most people believe they are always hard to bake rather than fried.

When you toast the breadcrumbs, it makes all the difference because fish cooks so much faster in the oven than it takes to brown the breadcrumbs. It's a mess-free breading method.

PREP TIME: 15 mins
YIELD: 1 serving
COOK TIME: 15 mins
TOTAL TIME: 30 mins

NUTRITIONAL INFO

Calories: 266 cal | **Total fat:** 11 g | **Sugar:** 9 g | **Iron:** 1 mg | **Cholesterol:** 120 mg | **Carbohydrates:** 12 g | **Protein:** 35 g | **Fiber:** 1 g | **Calcium:** 77 mg | **Sodium:** 538 mg

INGREDIENTS

- Oil spray (olive oil or any plain)
- 150grams / 0.3 pound of white fish fillets, patted dry

CRUMB
- 0.5 teaspoon of paprika, optional
- 0.13 teaspoon of salt and pepper
- 0.38 cups (18.75g) of panko breadcrumbs
- 0.06 cup (6.25g) of parmesan

BATTER
- 0.5 tablespoon of flour
- 0.06 teaspoon of salt and pepper
- 0.25 egg
- 0.25 tablespoon of mayonnaise

SERVING
- Finely chopped chives or parsley, garnish (optional)
- Tartare sauce or other seafood dipping sauce
- Lemon wedges

DIRECTIONS

- Preheat oven to 180 degrees C.
  Crumbling:
- Toast breadcrumbs by spreading breadcrumbs on the tray.
- Spray with oil and bake until golden for about 4 minutes.
- Transfer toasted breadcrumbs into the bowl and add the rest of the crumb ingredients and mix.
- Increase oven to 220 degrees C and spray your used tray with oil.
- **For the batter:** In a separate bowl, mix all of the ingredients.
- Cut the fish into strips.
- Place the fish in batter and mix to coat using rubber spatula - don't around. Just coat immediately.
- **Breading:** Use tongs to pick up the fish and place into breadcrumbs.
- Spoon over crumb using your fingers to press to adhere.
- **Baking:** Transfer into the baking tray.
- Spray with oil, bake until crispy on the outside, for about 13 minutes.
- Serve immediately with lemon wedges. Enjoy.

Soups
Recipes

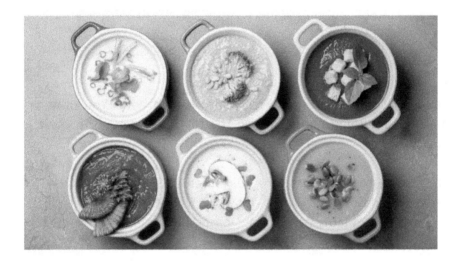

Adele Bayles

211

LENTIL SOUP

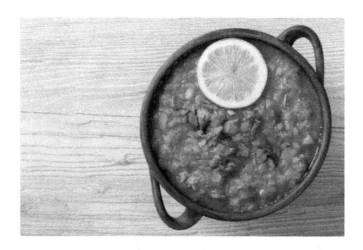

This is a one-pot lentil soup you would want to make. You know that making something nourishing on the table fast would be great for your health.

This recipe requires just ten (10) ingredients and can be ready to serve within 30 minutes. It's a lovely recipe that starts with hearty vegetables for plenty of rich plant-based fiber and flavor.

PREP TIME: 10 mins
COOK TIME: 30 mins
TOTAL TIME: 40 mins
YIELD: 1 serving

NUTRITIONAL INFO

Calories: 359 cal | **Total fat:** 2.7 g | **Sugar:** 11 g | **Iron:** 5.4 mg | **Cholesterol:** 0 mg | **Carbohydrates:** 68.7 g | **Protein:** 18.6 g | **Fiber:** 13.6 g | **Calcium:** 130 mg | **Sodium:** 764 mg

INGREDIENTS

SOUP

- 1 stalk celery, thinly sliced
- 0.06 teaspoon each sea salt and black pepper (divided / plus more to taste)
- 0.75 cups of yellow or red baby potatoes (roughly chopped into bite-size pieces)
- 1 cups of vegetable broth (plus more as needed)
- 0.5 tablespoon of water (or sub oil of choice / such as avocado or coconut)
- 0.5 cloves garlic minced (or sub 2 tablespoons of garlic-infused oil)
- 0.5 small shallots (1/2 white onion, diced - optional)
- 1 large carrot, thinly sliced
- 0.5-0.75 sprigs of fresh rosemary or thyme (you can use a bit of both)
- 0.25 cup of uncooked green or brown lentils (thoroughly rinsed and drained)

DIRECTIONS

- Heat a large pot over medium heat.
- Add water or oil once hot, shallots or onions, garlic, celery, and carrots.
- Season with a bit of pepper and salt. Stir.
- Sauté until golden brown and slightly tender, for about 4 minutes.
- Do not burn the garlic.
- Add potatoes and season with little pepper and salt.
- Stir and cook for about 2 mins more.
- Add rosemary or thyme and broth. Increase heat to medium-high.
- Bring to a rolling simmer. Then add the lentils. Stir.
- Reduce heat to low once simmering again.
- Simmer uncovered until lentils and potatoes are tender, for about 20 minutes.
- Add the greens, stir, then cover.
- Cook for 4 minutes more.
- Then taste and adjust if needed by adding more

- 0.5 cups of chopped sturdy greens (such as kale or collard greens)
FOR SERVING optional
- Fresh parsley

- pepper and salt for overall flavor.
- Serve with fresh parsley and enjoy.

KALE WITH BEAN SOUP

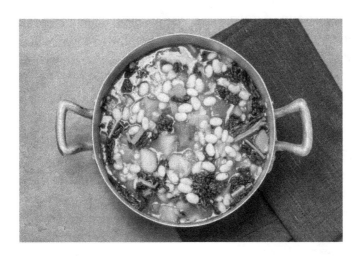

This is a tasty soup that uses fresh carrots and would be good with some pasta as well. You'll love the amount of garlic and even upped it.

Throw a dash of soy for umami and some red pepper flakes. This is a good combo vegetable and flavor combo. You can play around with it.

PREP TIME: 10 mins
COOK TIME: 15 mins
TOTAL TIME: 25 mins
YIELD: 1 serving

NUTRITIONAL INFO

Calories: 214.6 cal | **Total fat:** 2.7 g | **Sugar:** 3.8 g | **Iron:** 10.6 mg | **Cholesterol:** 0 mg | **Carbohydrates:** 36 g | **Protein:** 11.6 g | **Fiber:** 11 g | **Calcium:** 0 mg | **Sodium:** 786 mg

INGREDIENTS

- 1/4 teaspoon of Italian herb seasoning
- 1/8 to taste salt and pepper
- 2 (1 7/8 ounce) cans of sliced carrots, undrained
- 1 (3 1/2 ounce) can of diced tomatoes
- 1/8 cup of chopped parsley
- 1/8 to taste shredded Parmesan cheese
- 1/8 tablespoon of olive oil
- 1 garlic cloves, minced
- 1/8 medium yellow onion, chopped
- 1/2 cup of raw kale, chopped
- 1/2 cup of chicken broth or 1/2 cup of vegetable broth, divided
- 2 (1 7/8 ounce) cans of cannellini beans or (1 7/8 ounce) cans of navy beans, undrained, split

DIRECTIONS

- Heat olive oil in a large pot.
- Add onion and garlic, saute until onion is transparent and soft.
- Wash the kale, leave small droplets of water.
- Sauté, stirring, for about 15 minutes, until wilted and a lovely emerald green.
- Add 1/2 of the broth, 1 cup of beans (reserve 1 cup), all of the carrots, tomatoes, salt, herbs, and pepper.
- Simmer for about 5 minutes.
- Mix your reserved beans and broth until smooth in a food processor.
- Stir into the soup to thicken it.
- Simmer for 15 minutes.
- Ladle into bowls. Sprinkle with shredded Parmesan and chopped parsley.
- Serve with a lot of crusty bread.
- Enjoy.

BROCCOLI COURGETTE SOUP

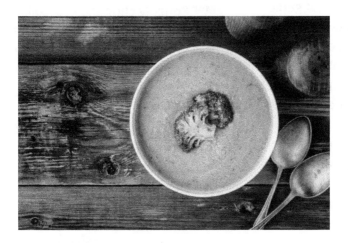

This green broccoli soup brings together courgette, onion, broccoli, olive oil, garlic, Parmesan, and water, and perform your magic.

This soup is so excellent for dinner.

PREP TIME: 10 mins
COOK TIME: 20 mins
TOTAL TIME: 30 mins
YIELD: 1 serving

NUTRITIONAL INFO

Calories: 214.6 cal | Total fat: 2.7 g | Sugar: 3.8 g | Iron: 10.6 mg | Cholesterol: 0 mg | Carbohydrates: 36 g | Protein: 11.6 g | Fiber: 11 g | Calcium: 0 mg | Sodium: 786 mg

INGREDIENTS

- 3grams of garlic
- 1/2 tablespoon of olive oil
- 225ml of water
- 40grams of parmesan
- 150grams of courgette
- 150grams of broccoli
- 90grams of onion

DIRECTIONS

- Roughly chop the broccoli, garlic, onion, and courgettes.
- In a saucepan, gently fry the chopped onion with the oil and garlic until the onion softens.
- Add stock made up with the broccoli, water, and courgettes.
- Heat till boiling, then turn down the heat and simmer until the vegetables are tender for about 10 minutes.
- Take off the heat and add the grated parmesan.
- Season to taste. Col a bit then put in the blender until creamy and smooth.
- Return to the pan to heat and add a bit more stock if you feel like.
- Serve and enjoy.

CARROT AND PUMPKIN SOUP

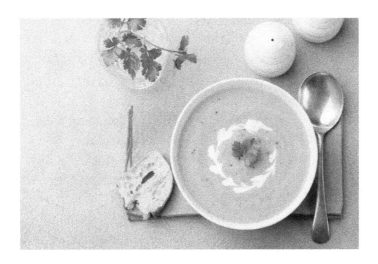

This is the kind of soup you should go for when the cold weather hits load your body up with flu and severe fighting. This soup is packed with all these tasty belly-warming carrot and pumpkin soup. It also features

Superfoods like garlic, turmeric, and ginger. It's a perfect meal you can eat in a bowl. It's so delicious as well.

PREP TIME: 10 mins
COOK TIME: 30 mins
TOTAL TIME: 40 mins
YIELD: 1 serving

NUTRITIONAL INFO

Calories: 190 cal | **Total fat:** 1.2 g | **Sugar:** 9.6 g | **Iron:** 0 mg | **Cholesterol:** 0 mg | **Carbohydrates:** 36.2 g | **Protein:** 9.8 g | **Fiber:** 12.3 g | **Calcium:** 0 mg | **Sodium:** 0 mg

INGREDIENTS

- 0.17 cup of dried red lentils
- 0.25 large of vegetable stock
- 1.33 sprigs of fresh thyme
- 0.17 medium brown onion cut into thin wedges
- 0.5 cloves garlic sliced
- 0.83 large carrots roughly chopped
- 50 grams of kent pumpkin, peeled, and cut into 3cm chunks
- 0.33 tablespoon of avocado oil or extra virgin olive oil
- 0.17 teaspoon of ground turmeric
- sea salt and pepper to taste
- 0.33 teaspoon of freshly grated ginger
- Greek-style natural yogurt to serve

DIRECTIONS

- Preheat oven to 400 degrees F.
- Arrange garlic, onion, pumpkin, and carrots on a baking tray.
- Add turmeric and oil and toss well to coat.
- Roast vegetables until tender, for about 25 minutes.
- Pop the lentils while vegetables are roasting, stock, thyme, and ginger into a large heavy-based saucepan.
- Cover and bring to a simmer over a medium-heat.
- Remove the cover once simmering and cook uncovered until lentils are tender, for about 30 minutes.
- Add them to the cooked lentil mixture once vegetables are roasted and simmer for another 5 minutes.
- Blend the soup to a consistency of your liking using an immersion blender.
- Serve and enjoy.

CREAMY POTATO SOUP

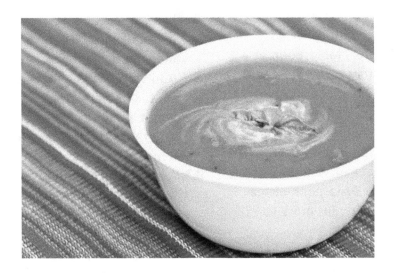

This is a Creamy Tomato Soup recipe. It reheats and freezes perfectly. This is the kind of recipe that can be ready-to-consume within 35 minutes.

This Tomato soup is such a comfort food for you. You can add it to one of your favorite treats.

PREP TIME: 10 mins
COOK TIME: 30 mins
TOTAL TIME: 40 mins
YIELD: 1 serving

NUTRITIONAL INFO

Calories: 208 cal | **Total fat:** 11.4 g | **Sugar:** 10.3 g | **Iron:** 0 mg | **Cholesterol:** 5.4 mg | **Carbohydrates:** 20.6 g | **Protein:** 7.7 g | **Fiber:** 4 g | **Calcium:** 0 mg | **Sodium:** 0 mg

INGREDIENTS

- 1.25 vine-ripened tomatoes, diced
- 0.25 tablespoon of tomato paste
- 2 fresh basil leaves
- 0.75 cups of low sodium chicken broth (or vegetable broth if vegan/vegetarian)
- 0.5 teaspoon of sea salt, plus more to taste
- 0.06 teaspoon of ground black pepper, plus more to taste
- 0.19 cup of unsweetened almond milk
- 0.5 tablespoon of olive oil
- 0.25 red onion, diced
- 0.5 carrots, diced
- 0.75 cloves garlic, minced

DIRECTIONS

- In a large deep stockpot, heat the olive oil over medium heat.
- Add carrots and onion and saute until tender, for about 8 minutes.
- Add the garlic and cook for a minute.
- Add tomato paste, tomatoes, chicken stock, basil, pepper, and salt and stir well.
- Bring the soup to boil and simmer on low heat, uncovered until the tomatoes are very tender, for about 30 minutes.
- Use a food processor, blender, or immersion blender to blend until pureed.
- Return to the pot if applicable.
- Add almond milk and stir to combine.
- Season to taste with any additional salt with pepper.
- Serve and enjoy.

SHRIMP GARLIC BUTTER SOUP

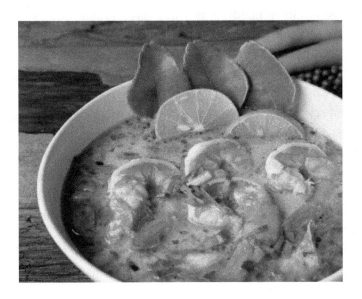

This recipe is easy to throw together and can be served over anything. This soup can be ready to consume within 15 minutes.

You can stir a handful of hair pasta through the garlicky, lemony, buttery sauce for a delicious dinner. This recipe should be found at your dinner table for at least once a week.

PREP TIME: 10 mins
COOK TIME: 10 mins
TOTAL TIME: 20 mins
YIELD: 1 serving

NUTRITIONAL INFO

Calories: 338 cal | **Total fat:** 18 g | **Sugar:** 0 g | **Iron:** 4.3 mg | **Cholesterol:** 540 mg | **Carbohydrates:** 1 g | **Protein:** 40 g | **Fiber:** 4 g | **Calcium:** 298 mg | **Sodium:** 1544 mg

INGREDIENTS

- 1 cloves garlic, minced (or 1 tablespoon)
- 0.44 pounds of (800 g) shrimp (or prawns), peeled and deveined, tails intact
- Kosher salt, to taste
- 0.08 cup of butter, divided
- Freshly ground black pepper, to taste
- Juice of half a lemon (about 2 tablespoons - add more if desired)
- 0.5 tablespoons of water
- Fresh chopped parsley, to garnish

DIRECTIONS

- In a large skillet, melt 2 tablespoons of butter over medium high heat.
- Add the garlic and cook for a minute, until fragrant.
- Fry shrimp and add pepper with salt to your taste.
- Cook for 2 minutes per side, stirring occasionally.
- Flip and cook until just beginning to turn pink on the other side.
- Add in the lemon juice, remaining butter, and water.
- Cook, while stirring, until the shrimp have cooked through and the butter melts.
- Reduce heat, taste it, and add more lemon juice, pepper, or salt, if needed to suit your tastes.
- Garnish with fresh chopped parsley or serve over pasta or rice.
- Enjoy.

SWEET POTATO SOUP

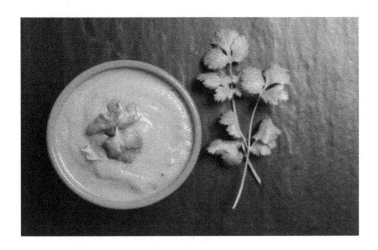

This soup is a rich blend of creamy sweet potatoes, fresh ginger, carrots, and a hint of spice.

It's very delicious, velvety smooth, and filling. Give it a try tonight!

PREP TIME: 10 mins
COOK TIME: 30 mins
TOTAL TIME: 40 mins
YIELD: 1 serving

NUTRITIONAL INFO

Calories: 254 cal | **Total fat:** 7 g | **Sugar:** 13 g | **Iron:** 1 mg | **Carbohydrates:** 45 g | **Protein:** 4 g | **Fiber:** 7 g | **Calcium:** 75 mg | **Sodium:** 1054 mg

INGREDIENTS

- 2 garlic cloves minced
- 1 tablespoon of fresh ginger finely chopped
- 1/4 teaspoon of red pepper flakes
- 1/4 teaspoon of paprika
- 2 tablespoons of olive oil or avocado oil
- 3 carrots sliced
- 1 yellow onion
- 1 1/2 pound of sweet potatoes diced and peeled
- 4 cups of vegetable broth or more for thinner consistency

Garnish
- red pepper flakes
- cracked black pepper
- watercress
- pistachios
- coconut cream or yogurt

DIRECTIONS

- In a large stockpot over medium high heat, heat the oil.
- Add the carrots and diced onion, then stir until the carrots have softened slightly, for about 6 minutes frequently.
- Add the ginger, garlic, paprika, and red pepper flakes.
- Stir until fragrant, for about 2 to 3 minutes.
- Add the vegetable broth and diced sweet potato.
- Turn the heat to high and bring to a boil.
- Reduce the heat to low and a lid, then simmer until the sweet potato is fork-tender, for about 15 minutes.
- Transfer the soup ingredients using a ladle to a high powered blender.
- Blend on high until creamy for a minute.
- You can add more water or broth for a thinner consistency.
- If you want to serve, pour into a bowl, then garnish with chopped pistachios, yogurt or cream, cracked black pepper, red flakes, and/or watercress.
- Enjoy.

TURMERIC SOUP WITH LENTIL

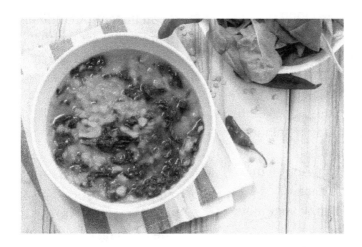

This soup is the kind of soup you can freeze up to about three (3) months. You can store in portions and let defrost overnight in the fridge. You can maybe, reheat in the microwave from frozen for about 6 to 8 minutes. Stir it halfway through the time you're heating it.

This is a vibrant, vegan, and delicious soup made with spices and coconut milk. Place everything in one pot, and your dinner is ready under 20 minutes.

PREP TIME: 20 mins
COOK TIME: 20 mins
TOTAL TIME: 40 mins
YIELD: 1 serving

NUTRITIONAL INFO

Calories: 418 cal | **Total fat:** 17 g | **Sugar:** 7 g | **Iron:** 0 mg | **Cholesterol:** 0 mg | **Carbohydrates:** 51 g | **Protein:** 19 g | **Fiber:** 22 g | **Calcium:** 131 mg | **Sodium:** 423 mg

INGREDIENTS

- 0.17 teaspoon of cumin
- 0.08 teaspoon of salt
- 0.08 teaspoon of pepper
- 0.25 cups of red lentils
- 0.67 cups of spinach, chopped
- 0.17 tablespoon of lemon juice
- 0.17 cup of vegetable broth
- 0.17 tablespoon of turmeric
- 0.17 tablespoon of olive oil
- 0.33 onions, chopped
- 0.33 carrots, chopped
- 0.5 stalks celery, chopped
- 0.67 cloves garlic minced
- 0.17 tablespoon of ginger, minced
- 0.33 (400mL) cans of full-fat coconut milk
- 0.17 (796mL) can of diced tomatoes (in their juices)

DIRECTIONS

- In an Instant pot, add all ingredients except for lemon juice and spinach.
- Make sure you add the lentils last.
- Cook on high pressure for about 3 minutes.
- It will take about 15 minutes for Instant Pot to come to pressure.
- Quickly release steam, by the opening lid when it's safe to do so.
- Stir in lemon juice and spinach.
- Then serve and enjoy.

HARIRA SOUP

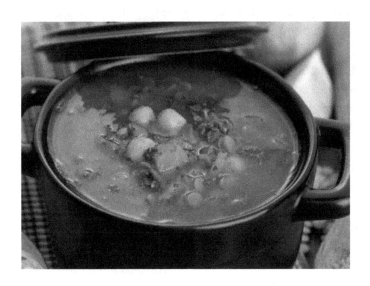

Harira is a soup from Morocco. If you want to make this soup taste good, you can season with pepper, salt, cinnamon, and mint leaves. I would want you to know that this is an excellent way to give your husband some good home cooking.

Enjoy!

PREP TIME: 10 mins
COOK TIME: 2 hours 30 mins
TOTAL TIME: 2 hours 45 mins
YIELD: 1 serving

NUTRITIONAL INFO

Calories: 467.4 cal | **Total fat:** 16.7 g | **Sugar:** 6.5 g | **Iron:** 6 mg | **Cholesterol:** 116.4 mg | **Carbohydrates:** 50 g | **Protein:** 29.4 g | **Fiber:** 13.3 g | **Calcium:** 85.7 mg | **Sodium:** 593.8 mg

INGREDIENTS

- 1/8 teaspoon of ground cayenne pepper
- 1 teaspoon of margarine
- 2 tablespoons of chopped celery
- 1/8 red onion, chopped
- 1/8 red onion, chopped
- 1 tablespoon and 1 teaspoon of chopped fresh cilantro
- 1/8 (29 ounce) can of diced tomatoes
- 1 cup and 3 tablespoons of water
- 2 tablespoons of green lentils
- 2-1/2 ounces cubed lamb meat
- 1/8 teaspoon of ground turmeric
- 1/4 teaspoon of ground black pepper
- 1/8 teaspoon of ground cinnamon
- 1/8 teaspoon of ground ginger
- 1/8 lemon, juiced
- 1/8 (15 ounce) can of garbanzo beans, drained
- 1/2 ounce of vermicelli pasta
- 3/8 eggs, beaten

DIRECTIONS

- Place the turmeric, lamb, cinnamon, black pepper, cayenne, celery, butter, cilantro, onion, and ginger in a large soup over low heat.
- Stir frequently for about 5 minutes.
- Pour tomatoes into the mixture
- Let it simmer for 15 minutes.
- Pour 7 cups of water, tomato juice, and the lentils into the pot.
- Bring this mixture to a boil.
- Reduce the heat to simmer.
- Let the soup simmer for 2 hours, uncovered.
- Turn the heat to medium high and place noodles with chickpeas into the soup, for about 10 minutes just before serving.
- Let it cook for 10 minutes.
- Stir in eggs and lemon.
- Let eggs cook for a minute.
- Serve and enjoy.

CARROT AND BEETROOT SOUP

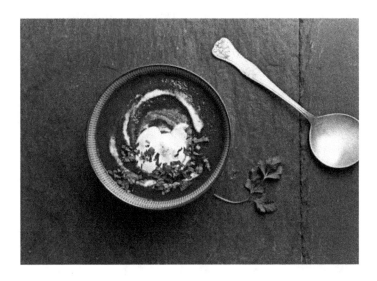

Carrot and Beetroot Soup is a vibrant, friendly, and delicious soup made with carrot, raw beetroot, and potatoes, garnished with crumbled feta cheese and cream fraiche.

Challenge yourself today to make this delicious soup. This soup is a comforting dinner soup you need to try.

PREP TIME: 5 mins
COOK TIME: 25 mins
TOTAL TIME: 30 mins
YIELD: 1 serving

NUTRITIONAL INFO

Calories: 206 cal | **Total fat:** 7.4 g | **Sugar:** 12.7 g | **Iron:** 1.9 mg | **Cholesterol:** 0 mg | **Carbohydrates:** 29.3 g | **Protein:** 7.8 g | **Fiber:** 6.3 g | **Calcium:** 170.6 mg | **Sodium:** 199.7 mg

INGREDIENTS

Soup:
- 2 garlic cloves, crushed
- 1-liter vegetable stock
- 1 tablespoon of tomato puree
- 2 bay leaves
- 500grams of raw beetroot
- 2 carrots
- 200grams of potatoes
- 1/2 tablespoon of olive oil
- 1 white onion
- 1/2 teaspoon of thyme
- salt and pepper to taste

Toppings:
- 80grams of feta cheese
- 1 tablespoon of parsley
- 2 tablespoons of cream Fraiche

DIRECTIONS

- Trim, peel and chop the carrots, beetroot, and potatoes into similar size chunks.
- In a large saucepan, heat the olive oil.
- Add the onion and fry for about 2 to 3 minutes.
- Add the garlic and fry for an extra minute just before adding the diced carrot, beetroot, and potatoes.
- Fry for 3 mins, stirring regularly.
- Add the tomato puree, stock, thyme, and bay leaves.
- Bring to the boil and reduce to a simmer until the vegetables have cooked through, for about 20 minutes.
- Blend the soup until smooth.
- Top with feta, cream fraiche and parsley.
- Serve and enjoy.

Snack
Recipes

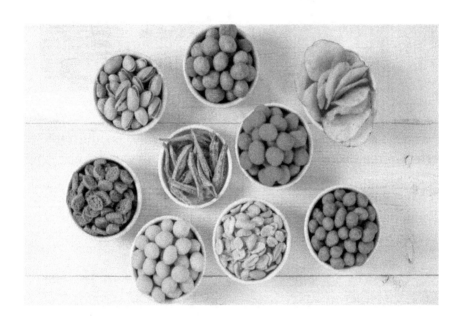

Adele Bayles

233

BAKING POWDER BISCUITS

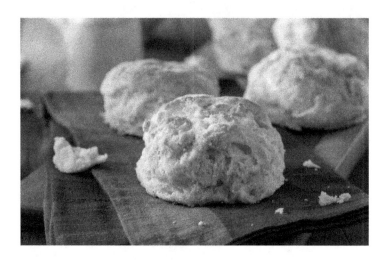

It would help if you had fresh warming biscuits on the table. It's perfect after taking the breakfast meal. It's as well savory supper and can be served with a cup of afternoon tea and jam.

All you need to do is mix a few simple ingredients, and in less than thirty minutes (30), you can have a delicious snack!

PREP TIME: 20 mins
BAKE TIME: 20 mins
TOTAL TIME: 40 mins
YIELD: 1 serving (12 biscuits)

NUTRITIONAL INFO

Calories: 160 cal | **Total fat:** 4.5 g | **Sugar:** 0 g | **Iron:** 0 mg | **Cholesterol:** 10 mg | **Carbohydrates:** 25 g | **Protein:** 4 g | **Fiber:** 6.3 g | **Calcium:** 0 mg | **Sodium:** 330 mg

INGREDIENTS

- 1 tablespoon (14g) of baking powder
- 1 tablespoon (12g) of sugar
- 3 cups (361g) of all-Purpose Flour
- 1 teaspoon of salt
- 6 tablespoons (85g) of butter, at room temperature
- 1 to 1 1/8 cups (227g to 255g) of cold milk or buttermilk (use whole milk for the most tender biscuits)

DIRECTIONS

- Preheat your oven to 425 degrees F with a rack in the upper portion.
- Bring out a baking sheet.
- Use parchment to lime it if you feel like.
- Weigh your flour or measure it by spooning gently it into a cup and sweeping off any excess.
- Mix flour, baking powder, sugar, and salt.
- Work the butter into the flour mixture by using your fingers, pastry blender, or a fork, a stand mixer, or a food processor.
- Your goal is an evenly crumbly mixture.
- Drizzle the smaller amount of milk over the flour mixture evenly.
- Mix for 15 seconds until you've made a dough.
- Don't keep working it if the mixture seems dry and won't come together.
- Drizzle in enough milk.
- Place the dough on a floured work surface.
- Pat it into a rough rectangle about 3/4-inch thick.

- Fold it into thirds and roll with a floured rolling pin gently until the dough is 3/4-inch thick again.
- Cut the dough into circles with a biscuit cutter.
- Place the biscuits bottom-side up on your prepared baking sheet, flipping them over. Bruise the biscuits with milk to enhance browning.
- Bake the biscuits until they are lightly browned, for about 15 to 20 minutes.
- Remove them from the oven and serve warm.
- Biscuits are always best when they are rewarmed before serving.
- Enjoy.

CHOCOLATE GRANOLA BITES

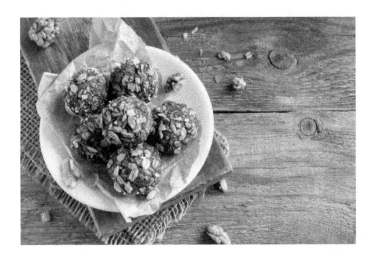

This is a sweet treat or a healthy snack for the lunch box. You can keep a bag of these awesome dark chocolate granola in the freezer or refrigerator.

Prepare this today and let it become a staple in your freezer.

PREP TIME: 5 mins
COOK TIME: 20 mins
TOTAL TIME: 25 mins
YIELD: 1 serving

NUTRITIONAL INFO

Calories: 100 cal | **Total fat:** 7 g | **Sugar:** 6 g | **Carbohydrates:** 11 g | **Protein:** 2 g | **Fiber:** 2 g

INGREDIENTS

- 1/2 cup of honey
- 1/4 cup of extra-virgin coconut oil
- 1/2 cup of creamy peanut butter
- 1 teaspoon of vanilla extract
- 2 cups of quick oats
- 1/8 teaspoon of salt
- 1/2 cup of unsweetened shredded coconut
- 1 cup of sliced almonds
- 1/4 cup of natural unsweetened or Dutch-process cocoa powder
- 1/2 cup of bittersweet or semisweet chocolate chips

DIRECTIONS

- Stir together the salt and oats in a large mixing bowl.
- Crush the sliced almonds into smaller pieces slightly.
- Heat a 12-inch skillet over medium heat.
- Add the almonds and coconut, stirring often to prevent burning and toast until the aroma is nutty and nuts, coconut is turning slightly golden, for about 5 minutes.
- Toss the mixture with the oats.
- Combine the honey, cocoa powder, chocolate chips, vanilla, peanut butter, and coconut oil in a medium saucepan.
- Heat the mixture over medium heat, stirring constantly, until smooth and melted.
- Pour the chocolate mixture over the dry ingredients and stir together until it's well combined.
- Scope the mixture into the tablespoon-sized mounds onto a parchment-lined baking sheet using a cookie scoop or 2 spoons.
- Let the mounds sit until they have cooked and are less sticky, for about 10 minutes.
- Roll the mounds into balls using firm pressure with the palms of your hands.

- Refrigerate the granola bites for about 1 to 2 hours to set up.
- They can be refrigerated for up to 2 weeks in an airtight container.
- Enjoy.

CHOCOLATE MUFFINS

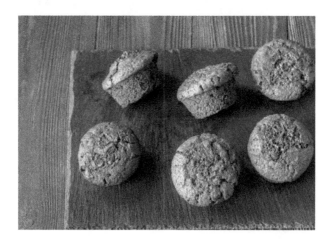

Chocolate Muffins are a delicious and moist snack that is full of chocolate goodness. It's even better when you keep for the next day.

This recipe is overflowing if you desire muffins so much. These muffins would be the best you ever had. It tastes luscious.

PREP TIME: 15 mins
COOK TIME: 20 mins
ADDITIONAL TIME: 1 hour
TOTAL TIME: 1 hour 35 mins
YIELD: 1 serving

NUTRITIONAL INFO

Calories: 321.6 cal | **Total fat:** 15 g | **Sugar:** 26.4 g | **Iron:** 2 mg | **Cholesterol:** 17.5 mg | **Carbohydrates:** 45.4 g | **Protein:** 5.4 g | **Fiber:** 2.6 g

INGREDIENTS

- 2 teaspoons of milk
- 1/8 teaspoon of vanilla extract
- 2 teaspoons of vegetable oil
- 1 teaspoon of chocolate chips
- 2 tablespoons and 2 teaspoons of all-purpose flour
- 1 tablespoon and 1 teaspoon of white sugar
- 1 teaspoon of chocolate chips
- 2 teaspoons of unsweetened cocoa powder
- 1/8 teaspoon of baking soda
- 1/8 egg
- 1 tablespoon and 1 teaspoon of plain yogurt

DIRECTIONS

- Preheat oven to 400 degrees F.
- Grease about 12-cup muffin or line with paper muffin liners.
- Combine 3/4 cup of chocolate chips, flour, sugar, baking soda, cocoa powder in a large bowl.
- Whisk yogurt, egg, vanilla, milk and vegetable oil in a separate bowl until smooth.
- Pour into chocolate mixture and stir until batter is just blended.
- Fill prepared muffins cups 3/4 full and sprinkle with remaining 1/4 cup of chocolate chips.
- Bake in preheated oven for about 20 minutes, until a toothpick inserted into the center, comes out clean.
- Cool in the pans for about 10 minutes before removing to cool completely on a wire rack.
- Serve and enjoy.

PEANUT BRITTLE

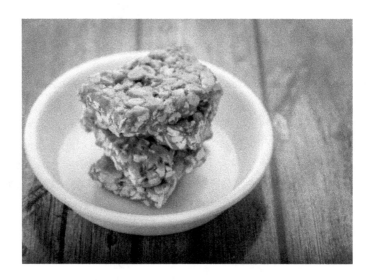

This kind of snack is soft on the inside and flaky with the slightest crunch on the outside.

There's nothing complicated about this recipe at all. They are mixed, cut, and baked in less than 30 minutes. The result would be the best biscuits you have ever eaten anywhere.

They are so crunchy. I love them!

PREP TIME: 10 mins
COOK TIME: 15 mins
ADDITIONAL TIME: 30 mins
TOTAL TIME: 55 mins
YIELD: 1 serving

NUTRITIONAL INFO

Calories: 163 cal | **Total fat:** 7 g | **Sugar:** 1 g | **Iron:** 1.3 mg | **Cholesterol:** 18 mg | **Carbohydrates:** 21 g | **Protein:** 3 g | **Fiber:** 0 g | **Calcium:** 69 mg | **Sodium:** 182 mg

INGREDIENTS

- 1/8 teaspoon of salt
- 3/4 teaspoon of water
- 1 tablespoon of peanuts
- 1 tablespoon of white sugar
- 1-1/2 teaspoons of light corn syrup
- 1/4 teaspoon of butter, softened
- 1/8 teaspoon of baking soda

DIRECTIONS

- Grease a large cookie sheet and set it aside.
- Over medium heat, bring to a boil sugar, salt, corn syrup, and water in a heavy 2-quart saucepan.
- Stir until sugar is dissolved and stir in peanuts.
- Set candy thermometer in place and continue cooking.
- Stir frequently until a small amount of mixture dropped into cold water separates into brittle threads when the temperature reaches 300 degrees F.
- Remove from heat and stir immediately in baking soda and butter.
- Pour at onto cookie sheet at once.
- Life using 2 forks and pull peanut mixture into rectangle about 14 by 12 inches, cool.
- Snap candy into pieces.
- Serve and enjoy.

SNICKERS BARS

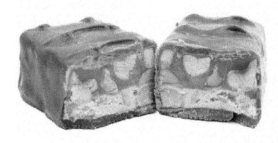

Theses Snickers Bars are two layers of chocolate, peanuts, creamy nougat, and plenty of caramel.

These homemade snickers bars taste just like the original candy bar. You have to melt peanut butter and chocolate together in the microwave. You've got this!

You would love them!

PREP TIME: 20 mins
COOK TIME: 20 mins
TOTAL TIME: 40 mins
YIELD: 1 bar serving

NUTRITIONAL INFO

Calories: 143.5 cal | **Total fat:** 6 g | **Sugar:** 15.6 g | **Iron:** 1.3 mg | **Cholesterol:** 0.2 mg | **Carbohydrates:** 3.8 g | **Protein:** 2.2 g | **Fiber:** 0.7 g | **Calcium:** 6.9 mg | **Sodium:** 132.2 mg

INGREDIENTS

- 0.08 cup of dry roasted unsalted peanuts
- 0.92 ounces of caramels
- 0.02 cup of heavy cream
- 0.17 cups of semisweet chocolate chips divided
- 0.25 tablespoons plus 1/4 cup, plus an additional 3 tablespoons of creamy peanut butter divided
- 0.58 ounces of marshmallow fluff
- 0.13 cups of confectioners powdered sugar

DIRECTIONS

- Line the bottom of an 11 x 7 inch baking pan with wax paper or parchment paper.
- Making the first layer:
- Combine 3 tablespoons of peanut butter and 1 cup of chocolate chips in a small bowl.
- Microwave for a minute at full power. Stir to combine.
- Microwave for some seconds if needed, until the chocolate is smooth and melted.
- Pour chocolate mixture into prepared pan and spread evenly.
- Place baking pan in the freezer for about 2 to 3 minutes until the layer is hard.
- In a medium-sized bowl, use a strong spatula or wooden spoon to combine 1/4 cup of peanut butter, marshmallow fluff, and powdered sugar, stir until a soft dough ball forms.
- Remove nougat dough from the bowl.
- Press on top of hardened chocolate layer.
- Sprinkle peanuts on top of the nougat and press them down gently.
- Combine heavy cream and caramels in a small saucepan over medium heat.

- Stir until caramels have melted and cream is incorporated.
- Pour it immediately over the peanut layer.
- Spread evenly using the back of a spoon and refrigerate for about 5 minutes, until caramel has set.
- Melt the remaining peanut butter and chocolate in a small bowl by microwaving for about 60 seconds.
- Pour over the caramel layer and spread evenly.
- Place in the fridge until chocolate layer has hardened, for about 10 minutes.
- Cut into bars using a sharp knife.
- Serve and enjoy.

PIZZA CRACKERS

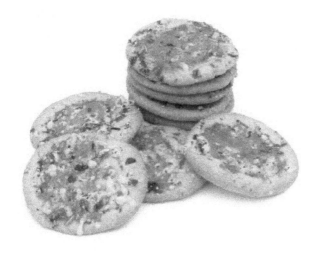

This is the most natural snack you can make with just four (4) ingredients. It's perfect for an appetizer, snack, or lunch for kids.

It's the kind of recipe you can easily change to your taste. You can make this recipe from start to finish in less than 10 minutes.

You can easily make more or less of these to suit your needs.

PREP TIME: 5 mins
COOK TIME: 5 mins
TOTAL TIME: 10 mins
YIELD: 1 serving

NUTRITIONAL INFO

Calories: 573 cal | **Total fat:** 20.2 g | **Sugar:** 69.3 g | **Iron:** 0 mg | **Cholesterol:** 6.8 mg | **Carbohydrates:** 97.9 g | **Protein:** 6.4 g

INGREDIENTS

- 10 thin slices of pizza pepperoni
- 1/2 cup of shredded cheese
- 10 Ritz crackers original, or mix it up
- 10 teaspoons of pizza sauce

DIRECTIONS

- Preheat the broiler.
- Use tin foil to line a baking sheet.
- Use nonstick spray to spray.
- And on a baking sheet, place crackers.
- Top each of the crackers with a piece of pepperoni
- Spread with about 1 teaspoon of sauce.
- Sprinkle with cheese.
- Broil until the cheese is melted for about 2 minutes.
- Serve immediately and enjoy.

BUTTERY PRETZELS

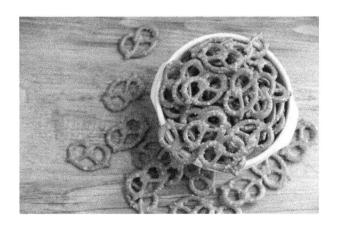

These pretzels are buttery and a bit sweeter than other types. Stop spending much money on those malls. You can make some for yourself seriously.

This recipe worked for me, and I'm sure it will work for you as well. These are vast plain with a bit of coated or pretzel salt packed with sugar and cinnamon.

Dip the hot pretzel in melted butter once finished and coated with your favorite flavors.

PREP TIME: 2 hours
COOK TIME: 10 mins
TOTAL TIME: 2 hours 10 mins
YIELD: 1 serving

NUTRITIONAL INFO

Calories: 42 cal | **Total fat:** 2 g | **Sugar:** 69.3 g | **Iron:** 0.2 mg | **Cholesterol:** 6 mg | **Carbohydrates:** 2 g | **Protein:** 1 g

INGREDIENTS

- 1/8 teaspoon of salt
- 1/4 teaspoon of vegetable oil
- 2 teaspoons of baking soda
- 1/3 cup of hot water
- 1/4 teaspoon of active dry yeast
- 2 teaspoons of white sugar
- 1/3 cup of hot water
- 1/3 cup and 1 tablespoon and 1 teaspoon of all-purpose flour
- 2 teaspoons of white sugar
- 1 teaspoon of kosher salt, for topping

DIRECTIONS

- Dissolve yeast in a small bowl and 1 teaspoon of sugar in 1 1/4 cup of warm water.
- Let it stand for about 10 minutes, until creamy.
- Mix flour, salt, and 1/2 cup of sugar in a large bowl.
- Make a well in the center and then, add the yeast mixture with oil.
- Mix and form into a dough.
- Add 1 to 2 tablespoons of water if the mixture is dry.
- Knead the dough for about 7 minutes, until smooth.
- Oil a large bowl lightly, place the dough in the bowl, then use oil to turn to coat.
- Cover with plastic wrap and let it rise in a warm place for about1 hour, until doubled in size.
- Preheat oven to 450 degrees F and grease 2 baking sheets.
- Dissolve baking soda in a large bowl in a cup of hot water, set it aside.
- Turn dough out onto a lightly floured surface when risen and divide into 12

equal pieces.

- Roll each piece into a rope and then twist into a pretzel shape.
- Dip each pretzel into the baking soda hot water solution once all of the dough is shaped.
- Place pretzels on the baking sheets and sprinkle with kosher salt.
- Bake in the preheated oven for about 8 minutes, until browned.
- Serve and enjoy.

BARK SNOWFLAKES

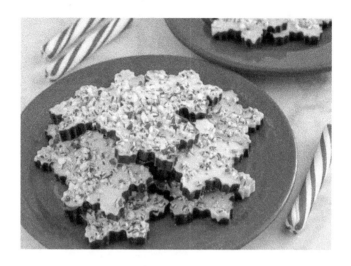

These Bark Snowflakes are perfect. They are so comfortable and simple to make. Melt white chocolate, add crushed candy canes, and peppermint extract.

This is an adorable and amazing wonderfully made Bark Snowflakes. It's just too pretty to eat.

PREP TIME: 20 mins
COOK TIME: 20 mins
TOTAL TIME: 40 mins
YIELD: 1 serving

NUTRITIONAL INFO

Calories: 237.1 cal | **Total fat:** 1.7 g | **Sugar:** 8.8 g | **Iron:** 2.6 mg | **Cholesterol:** 0 mg | **Carbohydrates:** 48.9 g | **Protein:** 5.9 g | **Fiber:** 1.7 g | **Calcium:** 12 mg | **Sodium:** 1422 mg

INGREDIENTS

- 2 teaspoons of vegetable oil, divided
- 1/2-1 teaspoon of peppermint extract, divided
- 6-8 candy canes, crushed into 1/4 inch pieces (remove dust)
- 8 ounces of white chocolate, chopped
- 8 ounces of semisweet chocolate, chopped

DIRECTIONS

- In a large microwave-safe bowl, melt 1 teaspoon of vegetable oil and semisweet chocolate gently. Stopping and stirring at maybe 30 seconds intervals till smooth and melted.
- Add 1/2 teaspoon of peppermint extract. Pout into your silicone molds.
- Sprinkle with some candy cane bits.
- Refrigerate when making the white chocolate layer.
- Melt 1 teaspoon of vegetable oil and white chocolate as you did the dark chocolate and then, add extract.
- Pour your white chocolate over the dark chocolate.
- Sprinkle tops with candy cane bits just before the chocolate hardens.
- Chill and then remove from molds to serve.
- Enjoy.

PEANUT BUTTER COOKIES

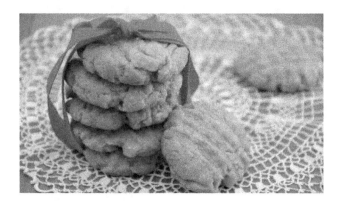

Peanut Butter Cookies are healthy, delicious, and a way to satisfy your cookie craving. With only five (5) ingredients, you can make this super easy treat for yourself. They are super great, low carb and sirtfood friendly.

They are utterly delicious and chewy. You can eat more than one without overloading on sugar. You'll be amazed at how easy and tasty baking can be.

PREP TIME: 5 mins
COOK TIME: 15 mins
TOTAL TIME: 20 mins
YIELD: 1 serving

NUTRITIONAL INFO

Calories: 474 cal | Total fat: 25 g | Sugar: 55 g | Iron: 0 mg | Cholesterol: 8 mg | Carbohydrates: 65 g | Protein: 4 g | Fiber: 2 g | Calcium: 0 mg | Sodium: 145 mg

INGREDIENTS

- 1 cup of smooth peanut butter (no added sugar)
- 1/2 teaspoon of baking soda
- 1/2 teaspoon of vanilla essence
- 1 large egg
- 2/3 cup of erythritol

DIRECTIONS

- Preheat oven to 350 degrees F.
- Use baking paper to line a cookie tray. Set it aside.
- Add the erythritol to a blender or Nutribullet, then blend until powdered. Set it aside.
- In a medium mixing bowl, add all of the ingredients and mix until smooth and glossy dough forms.
- Roll about 2 tablespoons of dough just between your palms to form a ball and then place on the prepared cookie tray.
- Repeat till the dough has been used.
- Flatten the cookies using a fork and creating a criss-cross pattern across the top.
- Bake the cookies for about 12 minutes.
- Remove from the oven.
- Allow it to cool on the baking tray for about 25 minutes and then transfer for another 25 minutes in a cooling rack.
- Serve and enjoy.

Dessert
Recipes

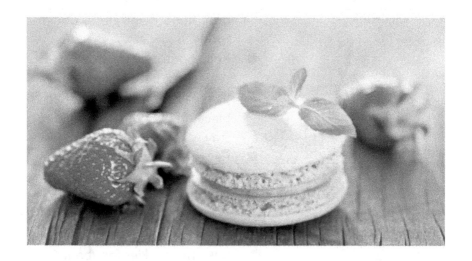

Adele Bayles

256

BLUEBERRY MUFFINS

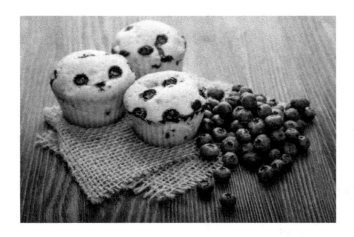

This blueberry muffin is loaded with sweet blueberries, plump and can be baked in a ramekin. It's got a beautiful and tender texture buttery flavor. You'll be glad to know that you're likely to find such a juicy blueberry in every single bite like this.

This must have a buttery taste and a tender crumb. It's easy to make and perfect size for a single person.

PREP TIME: 10 mins
COOK TIME: 15 mins
COOL TIME: 10 mins
TOTAL TIME: 35 mins
YIELD: 1 serving

NUTRITIONAL INFO

Calories: 693 cal | **Total fat:** 28 g | **Sugar:** 0 g | **Iron:** 3.6 mg | **Cholesterol:** 246 mg | **Carbohydrates:** 99 g | **Protein:** 12 g | **Fiber:** 3 g | **Calcium:** 182 mg | **Sodium:** 532 mg

INGREDIENTS

- 3 tablespoons of sugar
- 1 large egg yolk
- 1/2 teaspoon of vanilla extract
- 1/2 cup of all-purpose flour
- 1/2 teaspoon of baking powder
- 1/8 teaspoon of salt
- 2 tablespoons of melted butter
- 4 tablespoons of milk (or almond milk)
- 1/2 cup of blueberries

DIRECTIONS

- Heat oven to 400 degrees F.
- Mix baking powder, flour, and salt in a small bowl.
- Stir together sugar and melted butter in a separate medium-sized bowl.
- Add vanilla, egg yolk, and milk and whisk until completely blended.
- Stir wet ingredients into dry ingredients and fold gently in blueberries.
- Pour into a buttered 8 ounces ramekin.
- Bake until the top is golden and the center is completely cooked, for about 15 minutes.
- Remove ramekin from oven and then place on a rack to cool slightly.
- Enjoy with butter while still warm.

CINNAMON APPLE WRAPS

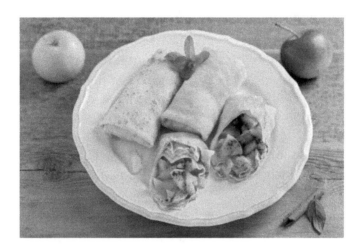

These beautiful wraps are a tasty dessert that is easy to make using tortillas.

It's a mouthwatering recipe and versatile as you want to make it.

PREP TIME: 15 mins
COOK TIME: 0 mins
TOTAL TIME: 15 mins
YIELD: 1 serving

NUTRITIONAL INFO

Calories: 442.2 cal | **Total fat:** 17.2 g | **Sugar:** 28.3 g | **Iron:** 0 mg | **Cholesterol:** 30.5 mg | **Carbohydrates:** 68.1 g | **Protein:** 6.3 g | **Fiber:** 5.8 g | **Calcium:** 0 mg | **Sodium:** 528.5 mg

INGREDIENTS

- 1 tablespoon of sugar
- 1/4 to 1/2 teaspoon of cinnamon
- 1 medium apple
- 1 tablespoon of butter
- 1 -2 tortillas (or wraps 8-10 inch size)

DIRECTIONS

- Chop the apples. But you'll have to peel it first.
- Melt butter in a small skillet.
- Sauté 1/2 of the apples in the butter with the cinnamon and sugar until tender but not mushy.
- Remove from heat, then add the uncooked apples, combining well. ;
- Place about 1/2 to 3/4 cups of the mixture on one side of each wrap.
- Fold over and then fold the sides in on top and then roll it up.
- Slightly press down and cut an angle into halves.
- Sprinkle with powdered sugar.
- Garnish with fresh mint.
- Serve with vanilla ice cream if you feel like.
- Enjoy.

STRAWBERRY MOUSSE

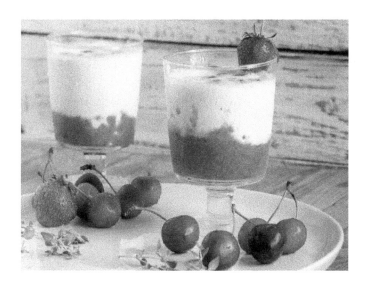

This Fresh Strawberry Mousse is a delicious dessert you can serve at any occasion. This is just a perfect fluffy mousse dessert made with only three (3) ingredients.

It's no-bake and no gelatin. It's easy and quick to make.

PREP TIME: 10 mins
CHILLTIME: 1 hour
TOTAL TIME: 10 mins
YIELD: 1 serving

NUTRITIONAL INFO

Calories: 330 cal | **Total fat:** 22 g | **Sugar:** 29 g | **Iron:** 0.4 mg | **Cholesterol:** 89 mg | **Carbohydrates:** 33 g | **Protein:** 1 g | **Fiber:** 1 g | **Calcium:** 53 mg | **Sodium:** 23 mg

INGREDIENTS

- 0.13 cup of granulated sugar
- 3.13 ounces of strawberries (3/4 pound)
- 0.25 cup of whole or whipping cream (cold)
- extra strawberries for topping

DIRECTIONS

- Clean and slice the strawberries.
- Add the sliced strawberries with sugar in a blender or food processor, then puree.
- Remove 1/2 cup of puree and set it aside.
- Add the cream in a cold bowl and beat until stiff peaks form.
- Then fold in the remaining puree gently.
- Top with the strawberry mousse.
- Refrigerate for an hour or over the night if you feel like.
- Top with fresh sliced strawberries.
- Serve and enjoy.

VANILLA ICE CREAM COCONUT CREAM

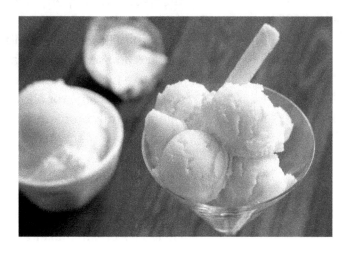

This version is quiet and straightforward, which possibly requires just five (5) necessary ingredients. What makes this recipe pleasant is coconut milk, vanilla extract, vanilla bean, sea salt, and organic cane sugar.

The extract helps prevent ice crystals, and the combination adds more flavor. The result is perfectly creamy.

PREP TIME: 10 mins
CHILLTIME: 1 hour
TOTAL TIME: 10 mins
YIELD: 1 serving

NUTRITIONAL INFO

Calories: 277 cal | Total fat: 22.1 g | Sugar: 14.3 g | Iron: 0 mg | Cholesterol: 0 mg | Carbohydrates: 17.7 g | Protein: 2.2 g | Fiber: 0.04 g | Calcium: 1.2 mg | Sodium: 34.8 mg

INGREDIENTS

- 0.25 14-ounce cans of coconut cream or full-fat coconut milk
- 0.06 cup of organic cane sugar (sub up to half with maple syrup or agave nectar)
- 0.13 pinch of sea salt
- 0.13 vanilla bean pod (split and scraped / or 1/4 – 1/2 teaspoon of vanilla powder per 1 pod)
- 0.25 teaspoon of pure vanilla extract

DIRECTIONS

- Place your ice cream bowl in the freezer to properly chill.
- Add organic cane sugar, coconut milk sea salt, vanilla extract, and scraped vanilla bean to a high-speed blender and blend on high for about 2 minutes until completely smooth and creamy to fully dissolve the sugar.
- Add more agave or cane sugar if it needs more sweetness.
- Add mixture directly to the chilled ice cream maker and churn according to instructions, for about 45 minutes.
- Transfer the ice cream into a large freezer-safe container once churned using a spoon to smooth the top.
- Cover securely and freeze until firm, for about 4 to 6 hours.
- Set out for 5 to 10 minutes before serving to soften.
- Serve and enjoy.

CHEESECAKE IN JAR

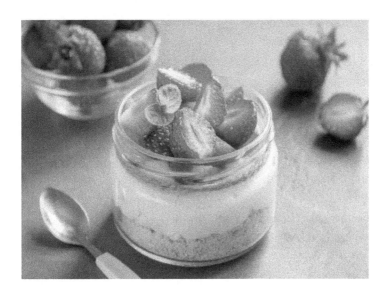

This recipe is packed with fresh strawberries, and it has a zero bake version of cheesecake in a Jar.

This cheesecake is so fluffy and light. It would be surprisingly easy to make, and everyone you share this with would love it.

Just follow this exactly and use blueberries, blackberries with golden kiwis. You would love it!

PREP TIME: 10 mins
CHILLTIME: 1 hour
TOTAL TIME: 10 mins
YIELD: 1 serving

NUTRITIONAL INFO

Calories: 412 cal | **Total fat:** 29.4 g | **Sugar:** 27 g | **Iron:** 1 mg | **Cholesterol:** 83 mg | **Carbohydrates:** 36.1 g | **Protein:** 4.7 g | **Fiber:** 1.1 g | **Calcium:** 57 mg | **Sodium:** 196 mg

INGREDIENTS

- 2 ounces of sliced fresh strawberries
- 1/8 (8 ounces) package of cream cheese, softened
- 1 teaspoon of fresh lemon juice
- 1 tablespoon and 1 teaspoon of white sugar
- 1 pecan shortbread cookies (such as Sandies), finely crushed
- 1 teaspoon of butter, melted
- 1 tablespoon and 1 teaspoon of white sugar
- 1 (1/2 pint) canning jars with lids
- 1 tablespoon and 1 teaspoon of heavy cream, whipped

DIRECTIONS

- Stir together butter, cookie crumbs, and 2 tablespoons of sugar in a bowl until blended.
- Divide mixture evenly among jars and press gently into bottoms.
- Garnish with maybe 6 strawberries and set it aside.
- Chop the rest of the strawberries.
- Beat together lemon juice, cream cheese, and 1/2 cup of sugar in a bowl with an electric mixer at medium speed until smooth.
- Fold in chopped cherries and whipped cream, then divide evenly among jars.
- Top each with 2 berry halves and cover with lids.
- Chill at least 2 hours or maybe 3 days.
- Serve and enjoy.

BLUEBERRY CHOCOLATE CAKE

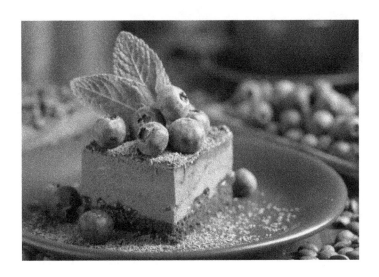

This Blueberry Chocolate Cake is a dark delicious, and dense brownie dessert. The idea of blueberries in chocolate cake batter is intriguing.

PREP TIME: 10 mins
COOK TIME: 30 mins
TOTAL TIME: 40 mins
YIELD: 1 serving

NUTRITIONAL INFO

Calories: 144 cal | **Total fat:** 1.2 | **Sugar:** 27 g | **Iron:** 15 mg | **Cholesterol:** 0 mg | **Carbohydrates:** 34 g | **Protein:** 3.6 g | **Fiber:** 4.4 g | **Calcium:** 0 mg | **Sodium:** 217 mg

INGREDIENTS

- 0.03 teaspoon of salt
- 0.09 cup of water
- 0.06 cup of blueberries
- 0.13 teaspoon of balsamic vinegar
- 0.16 cup of whole wheat flour (white whole wheat preferred)
- 0.75 tablespoons of unsweetened cocoa powder
- 0.13 teaspoon of baking powder
- 0.06 teaspoon of baking soda
- 0.13 teaspoon of ground flax seeds or chia seeds
- 0.06 cup of date syrup , maple syrup, or other liquid sweetener
- 0.13 cup of blueberries (for serving)
- additional syrup or agave nectar to taste

DIRECTIONS

- Preheat oven to 350 degrees F.
- Mix cocoa powder, flour, baking soda, baking powder, chai, and salt in a medium bowl.
- Combine 1/2 cup of blueberries, water, and balsamic vinegar and then blend until smooth.
- Make a well in the dry ingredients.
- Add the blueberry and syrup mixture.
- Stir until completely mixed.
- Pour into an oiled 9 inches round cake pan.
- Bake until a toothpick inserted in center comes out clean, for about 30 minutes.
- Cool completely before inverting onto a serving platter.
- Serve with blueberries on top.
- Drizzle with agave or syrup.
- Enjoy.

RED VELVET CAKE

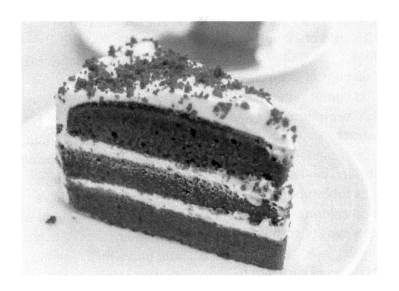

This recipe is the most amazing dessert I've ever tasted. This recipe is fluffy, moist, and it has the perfect balance between chocolate and acidity.

You can top this beautiful cake with some cream cheese. It tastes just so perfect!

PREP TIME: 20 mins
COOK TIME: 35 mins
TOTAL TIME: 55 mins
YIELD: 1 serving

NUTRITIONAL INFO

Calories: 411 cal | **Total fat:** 24 g | **Sugar:** 32 g | **Iron:** 4 mg | **Cholesterol:** 93 mg | **Carbohydrates:** 47 g | **Protein:** 6 g | **Fiber:** 4 g | **Calcium:** 41 mg | **Sodium:** 28 mg

INGREDIENTS

Cake:
- 0.19 cups of all-purpose flour
- 0.08 cups of warm water
- 0.03 cup of vegetable oil
- 0.06 teaspoon of vanilla extract
- 0.06 teaspoon of distilled white vinegar
- 0.13 tablespoons of red food coloring
- 0.19 cups of granulated sugar
- 0.03 cup of cornstarch
- 0.03 cup of unsweetened cocoa powder
- 0.06 tablespoon of baking soda
- 0.09 teaspoons of baking powder
- 0.09 teaspoons of salt
- 0.25 large eggs
- 0.09 cups of buttermilk

Frosting:
- 0.25 cups of powdered sugar
- 0.06 teaspoon of vanilla extract
- 1 ounce of cream cheese softened
- 0.06 cup of butter softened

DIRECTIONS

- Preheat oven to 350 degrees F.
- Butter three 9-inches cake rounds.
- Dust with flour and then top out the excess.
- Mix together sugar, flour, cocoa, cornstarch, baking soda, salt, and baking powder in a stand mixer using a low speed until well combined.
- Add buttermilk, eggs, oil, warm water, vinegar, vanilla, and food coloring.
- Beat on medium speed until smooth. This would take just some minutes.
- Bake until the cake meets the toothpick comes out clean, for about 30 minutes.
- Cool on wire racks for about 15 minutes.
- Turn out the cakes onto the racks and allow it completely cool before frosting.
- **Making the frosting:**
- Beat together cream cheese in a large bowl until fluffy.

- Use a stand mixer or hand mixer for best results.
- Add in vanilla extract and beat until combined.
- Beat in powdered sugar and 1 cup at a time until the frosting is smooth.
- Assemble and frost the cooled cake.
- Serve and enjoy.

ESPRESSO BROWNIES

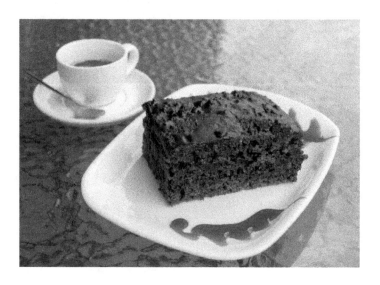

These Espresso Brownies are desserts that are made of fudgy, spongy, and loaded with indulgent and delicious coffee and chocolate flavor.

What makes the espresso brownies most delicious is the combination of these two things; Coffee and Chocolate.

PREP TIME: 10 mins
COOK TIME: 30 mins
TOTAL TIME: 40 mins
YIELD: 1 serving

NUTRITIONAL INFO

Calories: 657 cal | **Total fat:** 30 g | **Sugar:** 68 g | **Iron:** 1.9 mg | **Cholesterol:** 105 mg | **Carbohydrates:** 93 g | **Protein:** 6 g | **Fiber:** 1 g | **Calcium:** 86 mg | **Sodium:** 658 mg

INGREDIENTS

- 0.11 teaspoon of vanilla extract
- 0.33 large free-range eggs
- 11.11 grams of all-purpose flour
- 17.78 grams of unsalted butter
- 16.67 grams 70% of dark chocolate chopped into chunks
- 6.67 grams of ground espresso coffee (or about 2+1/2 tbsp espresso powder)
- 23.33 grams of caster sugar
- 0.33 tablespoon of organic maple syrup
- 5.56 grams of Dutch-processed unsweetened cocoa powder
- a pinch of sea salt flakes

DIRECTIONS

- Preheat the oven to 175 degrees C.
- Spray with oil one 8-inch square pan and use parchment paper to line.
- Set the oven rack onto the middle shelf.
- Fold in the butter and dark chocolate in a large microwave safe bowl.
- Cover the bowl and microwave for about 30 seconds, stir the ingredients and melt for another 30 seconds, until fully combined and smooth.
- Stir the ground espresso and sugar coffee into the bowl with the chocolate and butter. Then add the maple syrup and vanilla extract.
- Whisk to combine all of the ingredients.
- Stir in the eggs, one by one, wait until each of the egg is fully incorporated before adding the next one.
- Add in the cocoa powder, flour, and a pinch of salt.
- Stir until the ingredients are just combined.
- Make sure don't over-mix the batter.

- Transfer the mixture into the prepared pan.
- Spread evenly, leveling out the top.
- Bake for about 30 minutes, then insert a toothpick into the center of the pan. The brownies are not done if it comes out very wet. But the brownies are down if it's just slightly wet.
- Remove the espresso brownies from the oven and allow them to cool on a wire rack.
- Cut them into squares and serve.
- Enjoy.

PUMPKIN ROLL

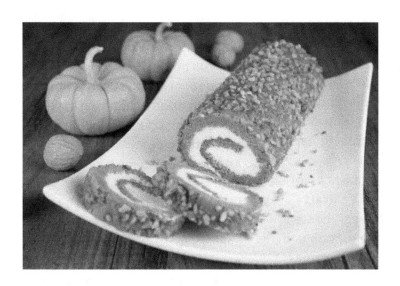

This pumpkin roll dessert is one of the most natural things you ever made. It's so easy, impressive, and delicious.

You might be a little afraid because of the whole rolling up a cake thing. I would have to say, do not be afraid at all. Its surely going to turn out to be very lovely and not too hard at all. It would be best if you can give it a try.

PREP TIME: 15 mins
COOK TIME: 25 mins
TOTAL TIME: 1 hour
YIELD: 1 serving

NUTRITIONAL INFO

Calories: 288.8 cal | **Total fat:** 11.8 g | **Sugar:** 36.6 g | **Iron:** 1.1 mg | **Cholesterol:** 86.9 mg | **Carbohydrates:** 42.2 g | **Protein:** 4.7 g

INGREDIENTS

- 1/2 teaspoon of butter, softened
- 1 ounce of cream cheese
- 1 tablespoon and 1-3/4 teaspoons of confectioners' sugar
- 1/8 teaspoon of vanilla extract
- 1/4 eggs, beaten
- 1 tablespoon and 1-3/4 teaspoons of white sugar
- 1/8 teaspoon of ground cinnamon
- 1 tablespoon and 1/4 teaspoon of pumpkin puree
- 1 tablespoon and 1/2 teaspoon of all-purpose flour
- 1/8 teaspoon of baking soda
- 1 tablespoon and 1-3/4 teaspoons of confectioners' sugar

DIRECTIONS

- Preheat oven to 375 degrees F.
- Butter or grease one 10x15-inch jelly roll pan.
- Blend sugar, eggs, sugar, pumpkin, and cinnamon in a mixing bowl.
- Mix baking soda and flour in a separate bowl.
- Add to pumpkin mixture and blend until smooth.
- Spread evenly the mixture over the prepared jelly roll pan.
- Bake 15 to 25 minutes in the preheated oven.
- Remove from oven and allow to cool enough to handle.
- Remove cake from pan and place on a tea towel.
- Roll up the cake by rolling a towel inside the cake.
- Place seam side down to cool.
- Prepare the frosting by blending the cream cheese, butter, vanilla, and confectioner's sugar.
- Unroll and spread with cream cheese filling when the cake is completely cooled.
- Roll up again without a towel.
- Wrap with plastic wrap and refrigerate until ready to serve.
- Sprinkle top with confectioner's sugar and slice with 8 servings.
- Serve and enjoy.

PECAN PIE

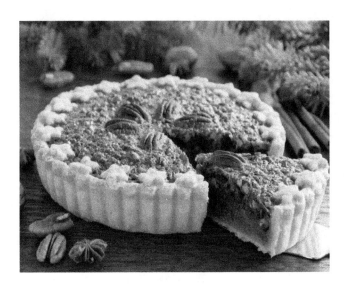

This is a wonderfully rich Pecan Pie you would ever try. It's undoubtedly going to be your favorite one, and this recipe is dynamite.

The result would either be a watery base and end up cooking the sugar mixture longer. It would make a big difference, and it's going to be exactly different from what you are looking for.

PREP TIME: 10 mins
COOK TIME: 1 hour
TOTAL TIME: 1 hour 10 mins
YIELD: 1 serving

NUTRITIONAL INFO

Calories: 511.8 cal | **Total fat:** 27.3 g | **Sugar:** 47.4 g | **Iron:** 1.4 mg | **Cholesterol:** 87 mg | **Carbohydrates:** 65.1 g | **Protein:** 5.4 g | **Fiber:** 2.5 g | **Calcium:** 28.2 mg | **Sodium:** 247.2 mg

INGREDIENTS

- 1/4 teaspoon of cornstarch
- 3/8 eggs
- 1/8 teaspoon of salt
- 1/8 teaspoon of vanilla extract
- 3 tablespoons and 1-1/2 teaspoons of white sugar
- 1-1/2 teaspoons of dark corn syrup
- 1-1/2 teaspoons of butter
- 1/4 teaspoon of cold water
- 2 tablespoons and 3/4 teaspoon of chopped pecans
- 1/8 (9 inch) unbaked pie shell

DIRECTIONS

- Preheat oven to 350 degrees F
- Combine the corn syrup, sugar, water, butter, and cornstarch in a medium saucepan.
- Bring to a full boil and remove from heat.
- Beat eggs frothy in a large bowl.
- Beat gradually in cooked syrup mixture.
- Stir in vanilla, salt, and pecans.
- Pour into the pie shell.
- Bake in the preheated oven until filling is set, for about 45 to 50 minutes.
- Serve and enjoy.

Juice & Drinks Recipes

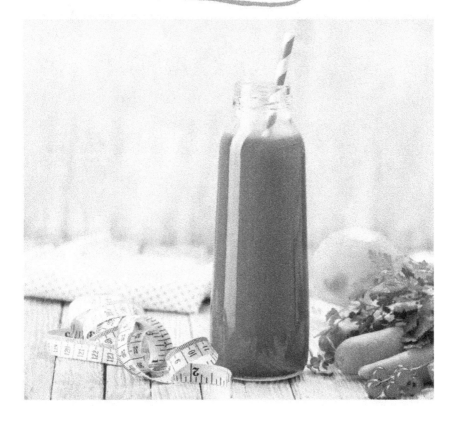

Adele Bayles

GREEN TEA MATCHA

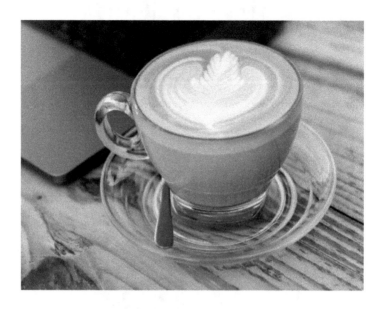

This Green Tea Matcha recipe is the kind of recipe that will energize you in an instant. This is a healthy blend of green tea, almonds, yogurt, spinach, banana, and kale all in one tasty sip.

This smoothie would give energy boost that you need to kick-start your mornings. It's effortless to add protein, fruit, fiber, antioxidants, and vegetables into your glass without compromising on flavor.

PREP TIME: 5 mins
COOK TIME: 0 mins
TOTAL TIME: 5 mins
YIELD: 1 serving

NUTRITIONAL INFO

Calories: 168 cal | Total fat: 4 g | Sugar: 17 g | Iron: 1.4 mg | Cholesterol: 2 mg | Carbohydrates: 31 g | Protein: 8 g | Fiber: 7 g | Calcium: 330 mg | Sodium: 140 mg

INGREDIENTS

- 0.5 banana, sliced
- 0.13 cup of sliced almonds
- 0.5 tablespoon of matcha green tea powder
- 1 cups of ice cubes
- 0.5 cup of unsweetened almond milk
- 0.25 cup of nonfat plain Greek yogurt, or dairy-free
- 0.5 cup of baby spinach
- 0.5 cup of baby kale
- 1 teaspoon of natural sweetener, Trivia

DIRECTIONS

- Add all of the ingredients together in a blender.
- Blend until the mixture is smooth, for about 60 to 90 seconds.
- Add more ice for a thicker smoothie or milk to thin the smoothie if you feel like.
- Serve and enjoy.

CELERY JUICE

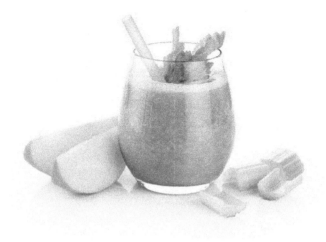

Celery Juice should be the first thing you need in the morning to activate and restore the gut, heal the body, and aid the liver.

This recipe would help you more efficiently and digest things faster. It also lowers cholesterol and lowers blood pressure. It has lots of benefits, and it's just so perfect for taking in the morning.

PREP TIME: 15 mins
COOK TIME: 0 mins
TOTAL TIME: 15 mins
YIELD: 1 serving

NUTRITIONAL INFO

Calories: 65 cal | **Total fat:** 0.7 g | **Sugar:** 5.4 g | **Iron:** 0 mg | **Cholesterol:** 0 mg | **Carbohydrates:** 12 g | **Protein:** 2.8 g | **Fiber:** 0 g | **Calcium:** 330 mg | **Sodium:** 323.2 mg

INGREDIENTS

- 1 bunch of organic celery

DIRECTIONS

- Use 1 bunch of organic celery
- Cut off the base to separate the stalks.
- Wash them in clean water to remove any debris.
- Chop the celery stalks into 1-inch pieces.
- Place them in the blender.
- Add 1/2 cup of purified water
- Put the lid on the blender and blend until smooth.
- Place a clean nut milk bag over the mouth of a bowl or pitcher.
- Pour the blended celery through the nut milk bag.
- Squeeze the celery juice using your hands through the bag.
- Drink immediately.
- Enjoy.

ORANGE KALE

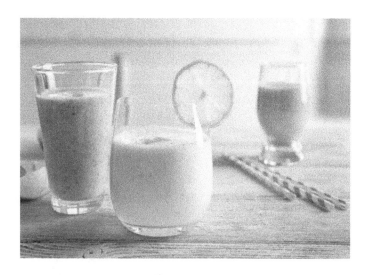

This recipe has less than five (5) ingredients and makes a perfect breakfast.

It's an excellent source of vitamins A and C, which may help support the immune system function and skin health.

PREP TIME: 5 mins
COOK TIME: 0 mins
TOTAL TIME: 5 mins
YIELD: 1 serving

NUTRITIONAL INFO

Calories: 130 cal | Total fat: 0.3 g | Sugar: 22 g | Iron: 0.49 mg | Cholesterol: 0 mg | Carbohydrates: 29 g | Protein: 2 g | Fiber: 1 g | Calcium: 0 mg | Sodium: 5 mg

INGREDIENTS

- 1 cup of kale, tough stems removed
- 4 mint leaves
- 2 cups of Florida Orange Juice
- 1/4 cup of frozen pineapple

DIRECTIONS

- Add kale, frozen pineapple, Florida orange juice, and mint leaves in a large blender.
- Serve yourself and enjoy.

CUCUMBER APPLE JUICE

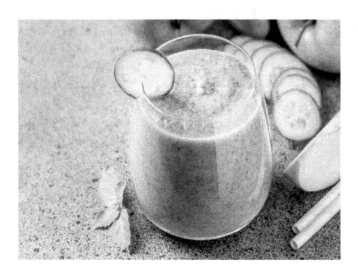

Cucumber apple juice makes a refreshing and light juice, which helps keep your skin glowing all day and detoxify it.

PREP TIME: 5 mins
COOK TIME: 0 mins
TOTAL TIME: 5 mins
YIELD: 1 serving

NUTRITIONAL INFO

Calories: 64 cal | **Total fat:** 0.5 g | **Sugar:** 0 g | **Iron:** 0 mg | **Cholesterol:** 0 mg | **Carbohydrates:** 14.1 g | **Protein:** 0.6 g | **Fiber:** 5.2 g | **Calcium:** 0 mg | **Sodium:** 33.7 mg

INGREDIENTS

- 3/4 cup of chilled and roughly chopped cucumber
- 3/4 cup of chilled and roughly chopped apples (unpeeled)
- 1/8 teaspoon of lemon juice

DIRECTIONS

- Add the cucumber and apples at a time in a hopper
- Add lemon juice to the juice and mix well.
- Pour the mixture into your glass.
- Serve immediately and enjoy.

GREEN LEMON JUICE

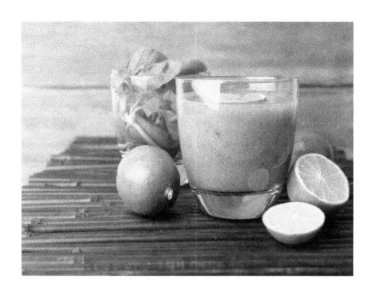

This Green Lemon Juice is made with romaine, kale, apple, lemon, and ginger, which makes for the most delicious nutrition and detoxifying drink.

It helps in preventing kidney stones and improves your skin quality. Also, it helps in promoting hydration in the body, and it's a good source of vitamin C.

Would you like to lose weight? Then, it would be best if you try this juice. So healthy!

PREP TIME: 5 mins
COOK TIME: 0 mins
TOTAL TIME: 5 mins
YIELD: 1 serving

NUTRITIONAL INFO

Calories: 158 cal | **Total fat:** 1 g | **Sugar:** 15 g | **Iron:** 2.7 mg | **Cholesterol:** 0 mg | **Carbohydrates:** 35 g | **Protein:** 7 g | **Fiber:** 6 g | **Calcium:** 238 mg | **Sodium:** 102 mg

INGREDIENTS

- 1 medium cucumber
- 1 green apple
- 1 lemon4
- 4 - 6 leaves of kale
- 1 head of romaine lettuce
- 1 medium carrot optional
- 2 celery stalks
- 1-inch piece of fresh ginger

DIRECTIONS

- Wash all of the ingredients
- Juice the ingredients just according to your juicer's instruction manual.
- You can use this method if you don't have a juicer.
- Sip slowly and enjoy.

WATERMELON JUICE

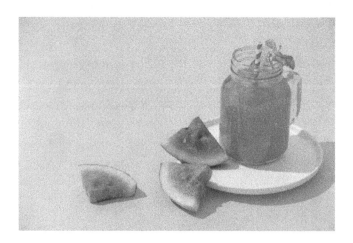

This kind of juice recipe is free from additives, and it's packed with nutrients.

A refreshing juice that helps in hydrating the body!

PREP TIME: 5 mins
COOK TIME: 1 min
TOTAL TIME: 6 mins
YIELD: 1 serving

NUTRITIONAL INFO

Calories: 114 cal | **Total fat:** 0 g | **Sugar:** 23 g | **Iron:** 0.9 mg | **Cholesterol:** 0 mg | **Carbohydrates:** 28 g | **Protein:** 7 g | **Fiber:** 2 g | **Calcium:** 1 mg | **Sodium:** 3 mg

INGREDIENTS

- 5 cups of watermelon cubes, deseeded
- 1/2 inch ginger
- 2 to 3 tablespoons of lemon juice
- 1 teaspoon of sabja seeds
- 8 to 10 mint leaves

DIRECTIONS

- If you're chai seeds or sabja, rinse them in a large bowl quickly.
- Strain into a coffee filter.
- Soak them in 1/4 cup of water for at least 30 minutes.
- Rinse watermelon under running water.
- Cut it to 2 halves and remove the seeds.
- Chop the watermelon pulp from the rind.
- You can chill the watermelon before juicing to avoid ice cubes.

Making the watermelon juice:
- Add the ingredients to a blender jar and blend till smooth.
- If you're using sabja seeds or soaked chai.
- Add then to your serving glass.
- Then pour the watermelon juice.
- Serve watermelon juice immediately.
- Enjoy.

VINAIGRETTE JUICE

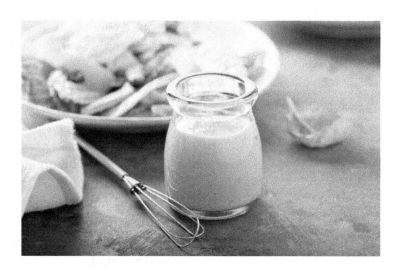

Vinaigrette juice is made with vinegar and oil and it's the easiest to whip together. As for the oil, you can go with extra virgin olive oil or avocado oil.

The avocado oil can be so delicious for this recipe. You would love it because it tastes so pretty.

PREP TIME: 2 mins
COOK TIME: 0 mins
TOTAL TIME: 2 mins
YIELD: 1 serving

NUTRITIONAL INFO

Calories: 180 cal | **Total fat:** 20 g | **Sugar:** 0 g | **Iron:** 0 mg | **Cholesterol:** 0 mg | **Carbohydrates:** 0 g | **Protein:** 0 g | **Fiber:** 0 g | **Calcium:** 0 mg | **Sodium:** 0 mg

INGREDIENTS

- 1 tablespoon of white wine vinegar (or balsamic, rice, apple cider vinegar, sherry, or other wine vinegar)
- 3 tablespoons of extra virgin olive oil (or a more neutral-flavored oil like grape-seed, vegetable or canola)
- Pinch of kosher salt
- A turn of freshly ground black pepper

Optional add-ins:

- 2 tablespoons of finely grated or crumbled Parmesan, Pecorino Romano, feta or Gorgonzola
- Pinch of crushed red pepper flakes, 1 tablespoon of horseradish, or 1/4 teaspoon of Sriracha
- 1 teaspoon of Dijon mustard
- 1/2 – 1 teaspoon of sugar or honey
- 1-2 tablespoons of fresh chopped herbs like basil, dill, parsley, mint, cilantro or thyme (dried herbs work, too, just use 1-2 teaspoons instead)
- A finely minced garlic clove
- 2 teaspoons of finely minced or grated ginger
- 2 teaspoons of finely chopped onion, shallots or scallions

DIRECTIONS

- In a small mason jar, add all of the ingredients.
- Screw on the lid and shake until blended.
- In a bowl, you can whisk the ingredients together or whisk them together in a blender.
- Taste and adjust seasonings if you feel like.
- Add to salad, toss and serve.
- Enjoy.

PINEAPPLE JUICE

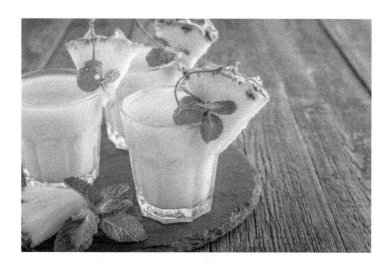

This Pineapple Juice is one of my favorite juice. Make sure you use ripe pineapples to make this.

Check out how to make it below by following the directions given.

PREP TIME: 5 mins
COOK TIME: 5 mins
TOTAL TIME: 10 mins
YIELD: 1 serving

NUTRITIONAL INFO

Calories: 121 cal | **Total fat:** 0 g | **Sugar:** 26 g | **Iron:** 0.4 mg | **Cholesterol:** 0 mg | **Carbohydrates:** 31 g | **Protein:** 0 g | **Fiber:** 2 g | **Calcium:** 19 mg | **Sodium:** 298 mg

INGREDIENTS

- 1 cup of Water
- 2 tablespoons of Sugar
- 300 grams of Fresh Pineapple
- 1/4 teaspoon of Black salt (Optional)
- Ice Cubes

DIRECTIONS

- Peel the pineapple and then chop it into small pieces.
- In a blender, add the pineapple pieces along with sugar and water.
- Blend to smooth the juice and strain the juice using a soup strainer.
- If the juice is too thick, add more water.
- In a serving glass, pour the juice.
- Add some ice cubes in the juice.
- Sprinkle black salt on top.
- Garnish with a pineapple wedge and mint leaves.
- Serve immediately and enjoy.

STRAWBERRY JUICE

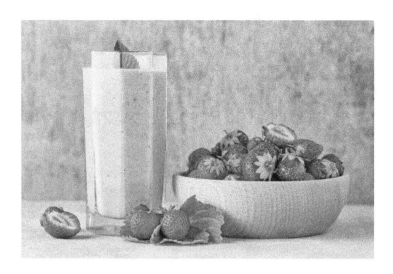

You will get addicted to this Strawberry smoothie. It's so simple, excellent, refreshing, and goes down so easy - you would appreciate the lightness of it.

Vanilla contributed to the flavor. It's great!

PREP TIME: 5 mins
COOK TIME: 1 mins
TOTAL TIME: 6 mins
YIELD: 1 serving

NUTRITIONAL INFO

Calories: 159.8 cal | Total fat: 1.1 g | Sugar: 29 g | Iron: 0.3 mg | Cholesterol: 4.9 mg | Carbohydrates: 30.3 g | Protein: 5.6 g | Fiber: 1 g | Calcium: 198.9 mg | Sodium: 71.4 mg

INGREDIENTS

- 1 tablespoon and 1-1/2 teaspoons of white sugar
- 1 teaspoon of vanilla extract
- 3 cubes of crushed ice
- 4 strawberries, hulled
- 1/4 cup of skim milk
- 1/4 cup of plain yogurt

DIRECTIONS

- Combine milk, sugar, yogurt, vanilla, strawberries in a blender.
- Toss in the ice.
- Blend until creamy and smooth.
- Pour into glass.
- Serve and enjoy.

BULLETPROOF COFFEE

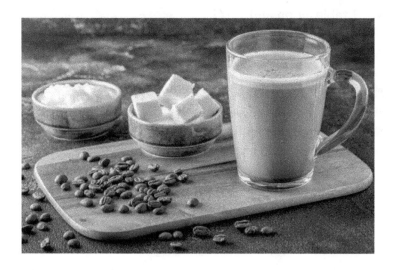

This Bulletproof coffee is a creamy, luxurious coffee fill with healthy fats. It's made with MCT oil, coffee, and grass-fed butter.

Do you want to lose weight? This is the best drink recipe you should go for. It will make your new morning fuel.

PREP TIME: 10 mins
COOK TIME: 0 mins
TOTAL TIME: 10 mins
YIELD: 1 serving

NUTRITIONAL INFO

Calories: 268 cal | **Total fat:** 29 g | **Sugar:** 0 g | **Iron:** 0 mg | **Cholesterol:** 76 mg | **Carbohydrates:** 0 g | **Protein:** 0 g | **Fiber:** 0g | **Calcium:** 0 mg | **Sodium:** 1174 mg

INGREDIENTS

- 12 ounces of Bulletproof Brewed Coffee hot
- pinch of pink salt optional
- 1/2 teaspoon of ground cinnamon optional
- 2 tablespoons of Ghee
- 1 tablespoon of MCT oil

DIRECTIONS

- In a blender, place all ingredients until fully combined and smooth.
- Serve immediately and enjoy.

7 DAYS MEAL PLAN

During the first three days of phase one, calorie intake is restricted to 1,000 calories. You drink three green juices per day plus one meal. Each day you can choose from recipes in the book, which all involve sirtfoods as a main part of the meal.

On days 4–7 of phase one, calorie intake is increased to 1,500. This includes two green juices per day and two more sirtfood-rich meals, which you can choose from the book.

MONDAY

BREAKFAST   Berries arugula salad (Pg.50) , and 1
               cup of Bulletproof coffee (Pg.298)

LUNCH   Chicken rolls with spice (Pg.101)

SNACK   Blueberry chocolate cake (Pg.267)
               and 1 Green Lemon juice (Pg.288)

DINNER   Chorizo potatoes (Pg.178)

TUESDAY

BREAKFAST   Kale omelet with smoked salmon
               (Pg.39) and Vinaigrette juice (Pg.292)

LUNCH   Shrimp with scrambled eggs
               (Pg.138)

SNACK   Peanut brittle (Pg.242), and Cumber apple
               juice (Pg.286)

DINNER   Beef rendang (Pg.203)

WEDNESDAY

BREAKFAST	Mushroom with kale frittata (Pg.45) and Pineapple juice (Pg.294)
LUNCH	Pork carnitas (Pg.105)
SNACK	Pizza crackers (Pg.247) with 1 cup of Bulletproof coffee (Pg.298)
DINNER	Nasi goreng (Pg.200)

THURSDAY

BREAKFAST	Coconut porridge (Pg.64)
LUNCH	Chicken curry (Pg.111)
SNACK	Buttery pretzels (Pg.249) with 1 cup of Strawberry juice (Pg.296)
DINNER	Teriyaki tempeh (Pg.190)

FRIDAY

BREAKFAST	Spinach with egg scramble (Pg.59) with 1 cup of Green tea matcha (Pg.280)
LUNCH	Shakshuka (Pg.124)
SNACK	Chocolate granola bites (Pg.237)
DINNER	Surf and turf (Pg.186)

SATURDAY

BREAKFAST   Sweet potato fries with avocado dip (Pg.72)

LUNCH   Basil with tomato sauce (Pg.180)

SNACK   Bark snowflakes (Pg.252) with Orange kale
                 juice (Pg.284)

DINNER   Fried fish vegetables (Pg.206)

SUNDAY

BREAKFAST   Swiss card with chickpea (Pg.66) and 1 cup
                 of Bulletproof coffee (Pg.298)

LUNCH   Cauliflower fritters (Pg.132)

SNACK   Snickers bars (Pg.244)

DINNER   Spicy meatballs (Pg.173)

TIPS: POPULAR QUESTIONS AND ANSWERS ON SIRTFOOD DIET

The Sirtfood diet is gaining popularity and followers just like, some well-known diet programs; the intermittent diet and the Mediterranean diet. As such, you might still have doubts and questions before you follow them. Answers to popular questions on the Sirtfood diet will be explained in this section.

FAQs for Sirtfood Diet

- Question 1:

How do chocolate bars, coffee, and red wine in weight loss; I thought those types of foods are unhealthy?

Answer:

Many people call Sirtfoods, 'wonder foods' but that is because they help people age better. Sirtfoods like chocolate, coffee, and red wine activate sirtuins that will boost metabolism rate, and this will increase the way you burn fats. An increase in the physical activity must always compliment the increase in Sirtfood consumption for better results.

- Question 2:

How many pounds will I lose after both phases of the Sirtfood diet program?

Answer:

Results vary from person to person. This is because of the different levels of commitment to diet, genetics, and environmental factors. But, an average person is expected to lose 15 – 20 pounds in the first three weeks. You could lose more if you restrict calories further but, that is not advisable because the whole essence of the Sirtfood diet program is for you to eat more Sirtfoods to activate sirtuins properly. Weight loss will be a result of that action.

If you plan to lose more pounds in 3 weeks (phase 1- phase 2), it is advisable to maintain the proposed diet intake of the Sirtfood diet program but, you should increase the intensity of your exercise routine. Push your body to limit every time you work out and the results will be mind-blowing.

- **Question 3:**

Is the Sirtfood diet vegan?

Answer:

No! The Sirtfood diet is not vegan. Some of the recipes in the recipe chapter of this book have meat and fish options. If the Sirtfood-diet were a vegan diet, those options wouldn't have been included.

- **Question 4:**

Is the Sirtfood diet gluten-free?

Answer:

Yes, it is! People who are allergic to gluten can follow the Sirtfood diet.

- **Question 5:**

Is it possible to increase the intake of Sirtuins activating compounds (SACs) without eating Sirtfoods?

Answer:

No, it is not possible. This is no approved pill or drug that will supply SACs effectively. The only way to get enough SACs is from a healthy Sirtfood diet. Peradventure, a pharmaceutical company, creates approved sirtuins modulators or pills; it will still be advisable to stick it.

DISCLAIMER

I am not a doctor. All information you read on the Sirtfood diet is only for educational and informational purposes. It is not intended for the diagnosis of any disease or undelaying health condition. You must understand that this book is not a substitute or alternative for any consultation with a licensed medical practitioner or licensed dietician.

If you still have questions on the Sirtfood diet, nutrition, and recipes, please do your research or contact your physician or health specialist. The author and publisher of the Sirtfood diet book will not be liable for any adverse reaction, effect, or consequences resulting from the use of suggestions, procedures, and recipes herein.

The publisher and author are also not responsible for any health or allergy needs that may require medical supervision.

All meal recipes in this book are tested. Still, there is also no surety that it will be turned out as described. Many things can affect how a recipe turns out – humidity, calibration of ovens, oven temperature, altitude, different climate, different appliances, various food sources.

Besides, there is no assurance that all opinions and facts in this book are the most recent because future medical research may impact all health and diet advice given in this book.

Lastly, there is no certainty about the success level after you have followed all steps and processes for the Sirtfood diet program. There is only about a 70% chance of success for anybody who will make the Sirtfood diet long-term. This is because any health-related program depends, but not limited, too; your capacity, genetic profile, life experience, patience, and commitment.

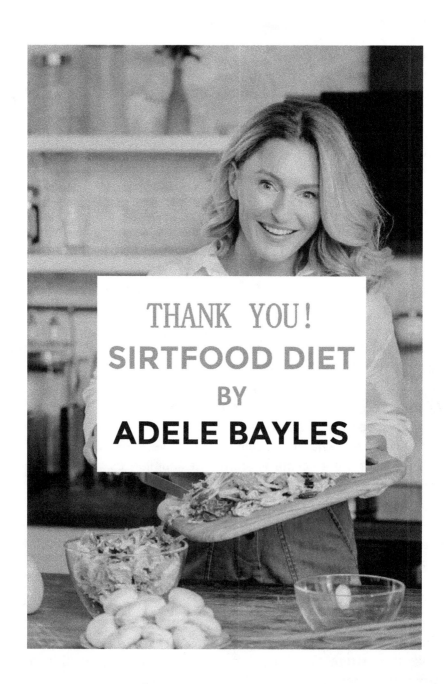

THANK YOU!
SIRTFOOD DIET
BY
ADELE BAYLES

CPSIA information can be obtained
at www.ICGtesting.com
Printed in the USA
BVHW080838091120
592842BV00007B/419